T0381970

Vegan Dairy

FIRST PUBLISHED IN THE UNITED KINGDOM IN 2019 BY
PAVILION
43 GREAT ORMOND STREET
LONDON
WC1N 3HZ

ORIGINAL TITLE: *VEGOMEJERIER*
TEXT © EMELIE HOLM AND NORSTEDTS, STOCKHOLM
PHOTOGRAPHS © JASON MICHAEL LANG
FIRST PUBLISHED BY NORSTEDTS, SWEDEN, IN 2018.
PUBLISHED BY AGREEMENT WITH NORSTEDTS AGENCY.

ISBN 978-1-91162-457-8

A CIP CATALOGUE RECORD FOR THIS BOOK IS AVAILABLE FROM THE BRITISH LIBRARY.

10 9 8 7 6 5 4 3 2 1

PRINTED AND BOUND BY 1010 PRINTING INTERNATIONAL LTD, CHINA

WWW.PAVILIONBOOKS.COM

THE PUBLISHER WOULD LIKE TO THANK FRIDA GREEN FOR HER WORK ON THIS BOOK.

NOTE TO READER: THE OVEN TEMPERATURES LISTED IN DEGREES CELSIUS WITHIN THIS BOOK
ARE FOR USE IN A CONVENTIONAL OVEN. IF YOU ARE USING A FAN OVEN, THESE SHOULD BE
DECREASED BY 20°C. BE AWARE THAT OVEN TEMPERATURES VARY BETWEEN APPLIANCES AND
ADJUST IF NECESSARY.

Vegan Dairy

MAKING MILK, BUTTER & CHEESE FROM NUTS & SEEDS

Emelie Holm

PAVILION

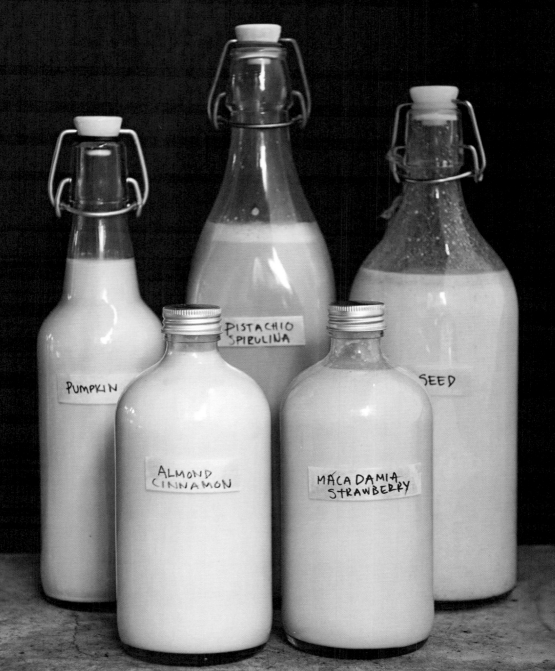

Contents:

My ambition with this book is to show how you can create your own vegan dairy products at home, rather than buy them in a shop. Buying ready-made almond milk might be convenient, but did you know that many brands only contain up to two percent of almonds? Moreover, nut milks often contain additives, such as thickening agents and preservatives, which many people would rather avoid. By making your own vegan milks, you will always have control over what you put into them.

With my recipes I want to inspire you, of course, and show how tasty vegan dairy products can be. The book is aimed at both beginners and the more experienced (yet curious) home cooks, who are looking for a greater understanding of vegan dairy. There are recipes for everything from quick nut milks to fermented products, including cheese and yogurt. There is also a chapter with ideas for breakfasts, snacks and treats where the vegan dairy products are either included in the recipe or can be served with your homemade nut butter or cheese.

It's easy to make your own vegan dairy. At the beginning of the book, there are details about which tools and kitchen equipment you need, a guide to different ingredients, and advice on how to soak nuts (and seeds) and activate them should you need to. There is also lots of useful nutritional information.

I wish you an enjoyable read and hope that you will be inspired to try making your own vegan dairy products at home.

Emelie Holm

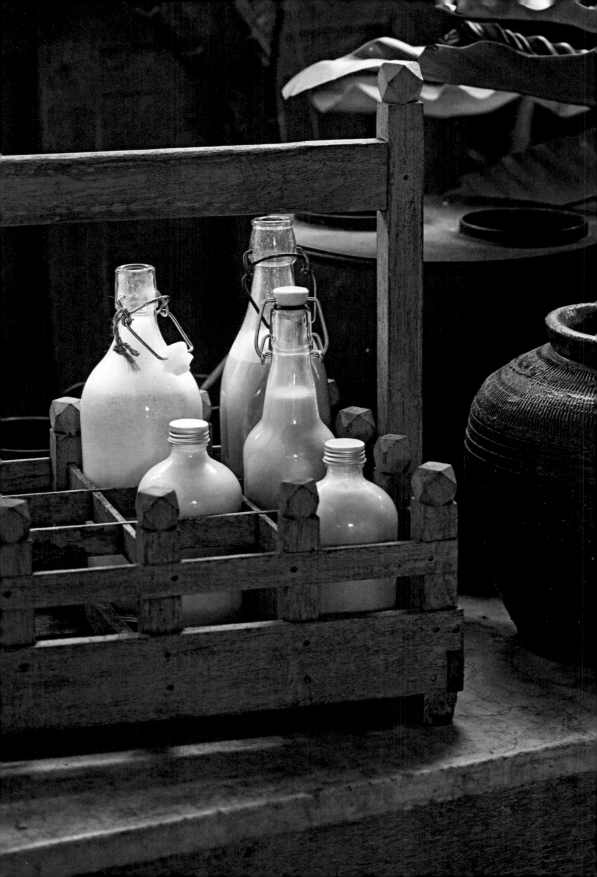

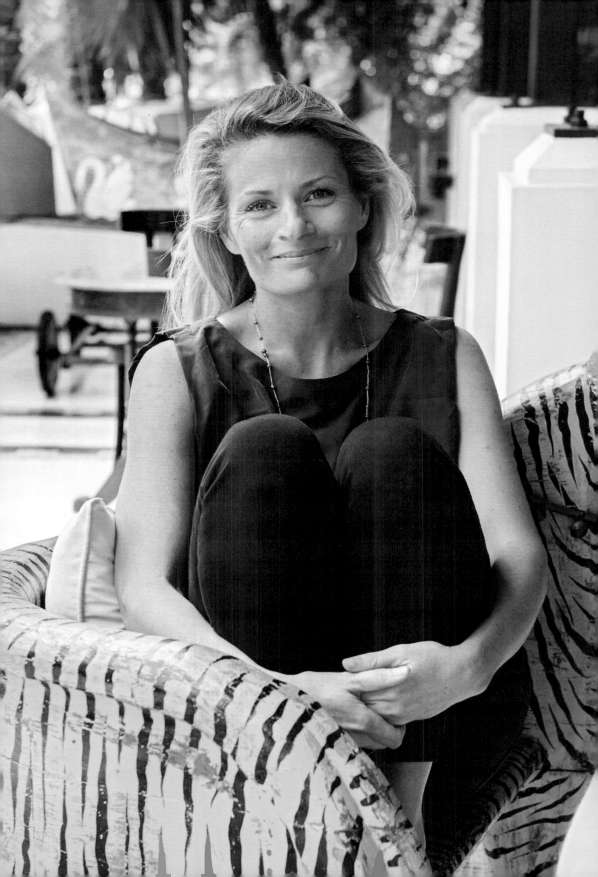

INTRODUCTION

The world is changing and so are us humans. When it comes to food, more and more of us are becoming interested in and more aware of what we eat and how it affects the environment, animals and ourselves. Vegan dairy alternatives have become a common sight on supermarket shelves and some people choose to quit cow's, goat's and sheep's milk products altogether. Some choose to give up dairy because of environmental reasons, others for ethical concerns – or alternatively simply feel better for not eating traditional dairy products.

WHY DO I CHOOSE VEGAN DAIRY?

Everyone has their own reasons for the life choices they make. For me, it started many years ago when I developed a greater understanding of how a large part of the food industry works and that it is sometimes enormously unethical. After that came the realization that the meat and dairy industry is also an eco-villain. But the decisive moment for me came when I felt that my health improved after excluding dairy made from cow's milk in my diet.

This is my third cookery book and in a way the end of a journey that I've been on most of my life. To feel good and to be healthy with a clear mind is the final destination, but also the start of a life with vision and plenty of energy. From a sugary existence with cupcakes and cakes, via baked goods without refined sugar to a life including wonderfully healthy vegan dairy.

I'm not going to lie, a life without animal products can sometimes be tough, especially if you live in a place where you simply don't have that much choice when you go shopping or eat out. The change is not easy, but I think it's worth all the effort once you have succeeded in breaking old patterns and routines. It's like taking up exercise: if you really want it, it will work. I actually have friends who always carry around some condiments when they go out to eat, just in case, so to speak… I've seen everything from pink salt, miso and tamari to avocado and dairy-free bread being pulled out of a bag at a restaurant!

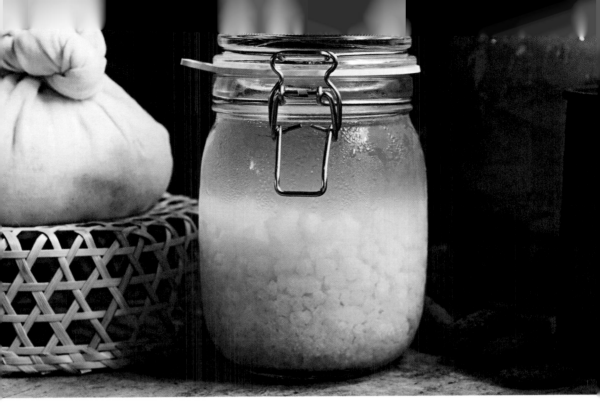

VEGAN DAIRY AND ALLERGIES

Natural unprocessed foods contain nutrients and healthy fibre that the body needs, but some of these foods can cause sensitivity or an allergy, and nuts are a typical example. In some cases, allergies that you've had since childhood can disappear once you're an adult. However, you can also develop allergies as an adult. I would recommend anyone who has a family history of nut allergies or suspects that they (or a family member) may have an allergy to nuts to consult their doctor before including nuts in their diet. It is also possible to have an allergy test at a naturopathic health clinic, but do check with your doctor first.

PROBIOTICS AND PREBIOTICS

Probiotics are beneficial forms of gut bacteria found naturally in certain foods, particularly fermented ones. They are also added to foods or are sold in supplement form, either in capsules or as a powder in varying strengths. These good bacteria survive digestion and contribute towards a beneficial atmosphere in the gut – otherwise called healthy bacterial flora – ensuring it is in balance and the digestive system works effectively. Probiotics also support the immune system.

Prebiotics can be described as the food that feeds the good bacteria in the gut and helps to increase levels to support healthy digestion. Largely, prebiotics are carbohydrates and certain types of fibre that the body can't digest or absorb, and these become food for the good bacteria instead. Prebiotics help the body to maintain a healthy gut flora and support thriving live bacterial cultures.

LIVE BACTERIAL CULTURES

Scoby and kefir grains (and probiotic capsules and powders) are all examples of live bacterial cultures. In order to ferment your vegan dairy products at home you will need one of the following:

– Scoby, which stands for symbiotic culture of bacteria and yeast. This form of yeast is added to sweetened cold tea, which is then left for at least a week to ferment.

There are two different kinds of scoby. One is for making kombucha, which is sweetened with sugar and is usually made from darker types of tea such as black tea and rooibos. The other is used for jun, which works well with light green tea and is sweetened with honey, although you could try experimenting with maple syrup or agave syrup. That said, if you want to make a vegan alternative of jun without honey, kombucha is probably your best option. Kombucha takes about 7–10 days to ferment, although it can be left for longer.

Kombucha or jun can also be used to ferment nut cheese and yogurt – you simply add a splash of the drink to the cheese or yogurt mixture and leave it to ferment.

– Kefir grains are used for making both milk- and water-based fermented drinks thanks to its bacterial cultures. There are two kinds of grains: one is used for water kefir drinks and the other for milk kefir drinks. Just like with a scoby, the kefir grains feed off the sugar that you've added to the drink, encouraging the fermentation process. Kefir is much quicker to ferment than kombucha or jun, taking about 12–24 hours.

Water or milk kefir can be used in the same way as kombucha/jun to ferment nut cheese and yogurt – just stir a little into the cheese or yogurt mixture.

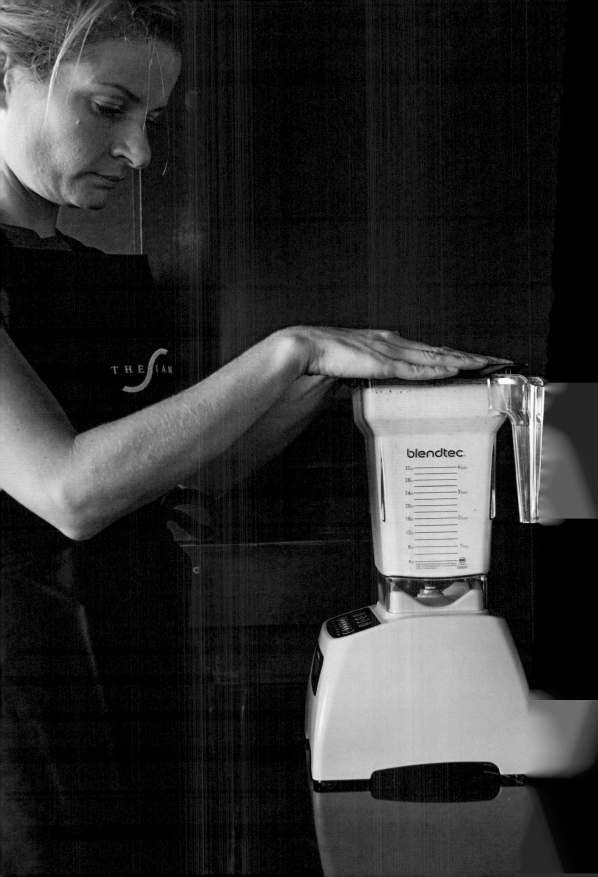

Water kefir

This is a good starter recipe if you haven't made kefir before.

500ml/18fl oz/generous 2 cups coconut water, at room temperature
2 tsp water kefir grains

Pour the coconut water into a sterilized glass jug or jar and add the kefir grains. Cover the top with a cloth or kitchen paper and secure with an elastic band. Leave to stand for 12–24 hours at room temperature until it looks and tastes slightly fizzy. Strain through a mesh strainer (not metal) to remove the grains. Pour the kefir into a clean bottle and store in the fridge for 2–3 weeks. (The kefir grains can be used again in the same way, although you may occasionally need to add sugar to feed the grains and encourage fermentation.)

– Probiotic powder or capsules (open them up to release the powder) can be added to your vegan dairy products and they work perfectly with everything from nut cheese to coconut yogurt. Both forms are easy to get hold of.

SUPERFOODS AND ADAPTOGENS

Most people probably know what superfoods are by now: not only foods such as fruit, vegetables, algae, seeds and berries, but also super-nutritious powders such as spirulina, chlorella, maca and acai.

Adaptogens are also plants and roots from nature, and they have been used for thousands of years in Eastern medicine. Examples of adaptogens include ashwagandha, liquorice root, rhodiola rosea and ginseng. They are included in a category of biologically active substances that, put simply, promote balance in the body. Adaptogens can help to restore and boost energy, increase focus as well as reduce stress and anxiety. Often available dried, the roots need to be soaked or cooked first to soften them. However, it is also possible to find adaptogens in more convenient powder or tablet form. I like to use both adaptogens and superfoods in my food. In the last chapter of this book, you'll find recipes where both are included.

TOOLS

Blender

If you are making nut milk you will need a good blender. It can be a fairly big expense, but you will thank yourself in the end. If you compare the price of a glass of homemade oat milk with a shop-bought alternative and then how often you buy it, you can quickly work out that it's an investment that pays off.

Food processor

The nut butter's best friend. Making nut butters can be a hard job for a food processor, even the flashiest of machines can tire quickly with the strain. Remember to let the machine pause from time to time and it will hopefully last for longer.

Dehydrator

A dehydrator is about the same price as a good blender. Personally, I borrow my neighbour's machine when I need to, so if you haven't got one, perhaps you can borrow someone else's? You can always bribe them with half of the batch of whatever you're dehydrating!

Nut bag/cheese bag

Straining nut milk or cheese is definitely easier if you use a nut bag or cheese bag, rather than a piece of muslin or a tea towel. I prefer a cloth bag, but if you don't have one you can easily make your own from a tea towel. A bag is needed to squeeze out the milk and also for covering cheese or yogurt.

Glass jars, plastic containers and bottles

If you don't have these at home you can easily buy them from shops or online. I use plastic containers for soaking, but apart from that I almost exclusively use glass jars.

Tape and pen

Always have tape or sticky labels and a marker pen at home so that you can label each container and keep a note of what you have made and the date you made it.

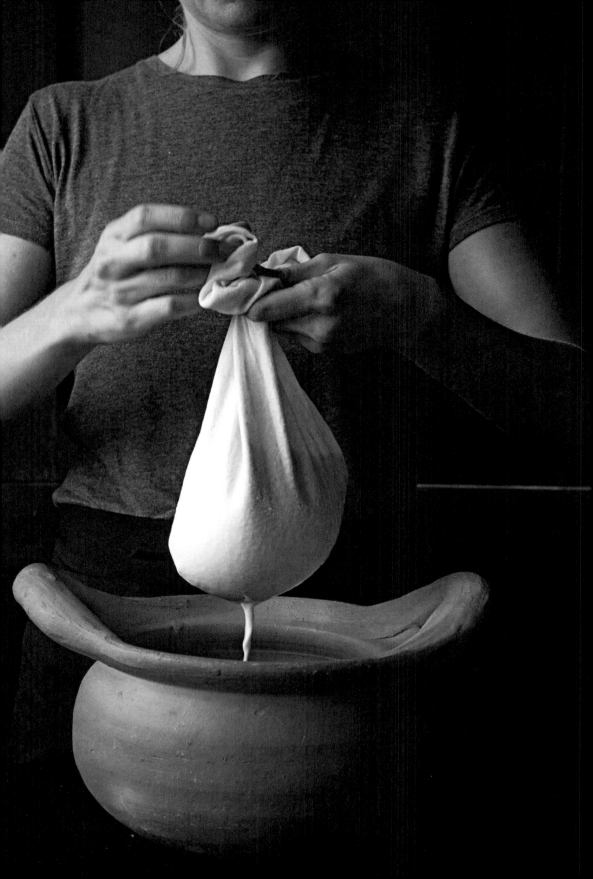

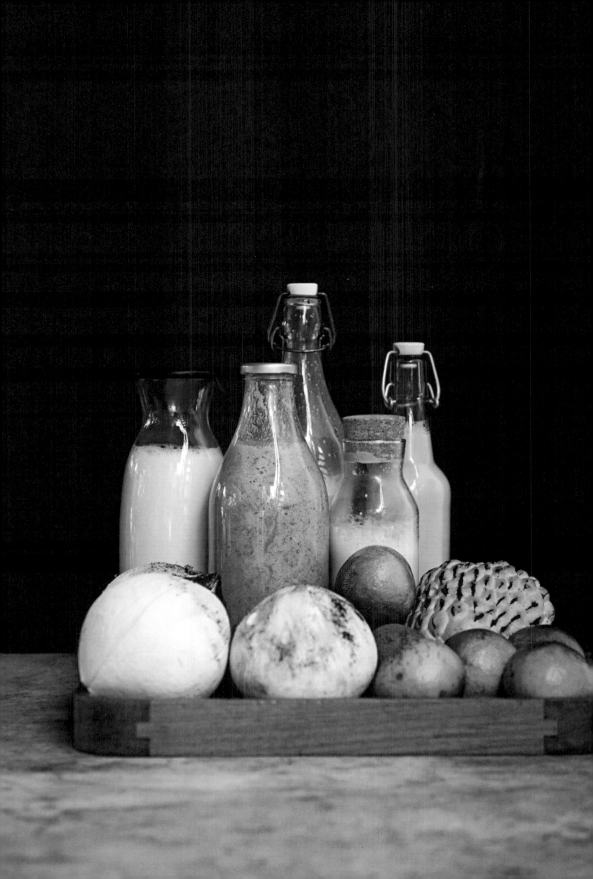

STERILIZING GLASS

When making your own vegan dairy products, jam or anything else at home that you store in a glass jar or bottle, it's important to sterilize them before use. Lids and caps need sterilizing too. This is to make sure that the food or drink keeps for longer and to get rid of any harmful bacteria and microorganisms that may spoil or contaminate the contents of the jar/bottle and make us ill.

Items that can't be sterilized in the oven such as metal lids with a plastic coating, plastic lids and rubber rings, can be boiled in a pan of water for 10 minutes.

How to sterilize

Preheat the oven to 140°C/275°F/Gas Mark 1.

Wash the bottles and jars, including metal lids, in hot, soapy water and place on a baking tray (sheet) in the oven for 10 minutes or until dry. If possible, fill the bottles/jars immediately, but if this is not feasible, make sure you don't touch the insides or the lids with your hands.

MORE TIPS

Freezing nuts

If you buy nuts in bulk, then it is possible to freeze them; this also goes for soaked or activated nuts. Raw nuts are perishable and turn rancid after a while which makes them taste bitter, so it is a good idea to put them in the freezer if you don't intend to use them within the date stated on the packet.

Plan ahead

Achieving a life free from dairy requires some planning – I'm not going to lie. Yet with planning comes a calming ritual to everyday life. There is nothing as calming as preparing thoughtful food, from soaking nuts to fermenting nut cheese – it's all rather pleasant, I promise! After a couple of weeks, once you've settled into your new routine, you'll notice that you don't want to be without your new life. And your calm, healthy gut will thank you too!

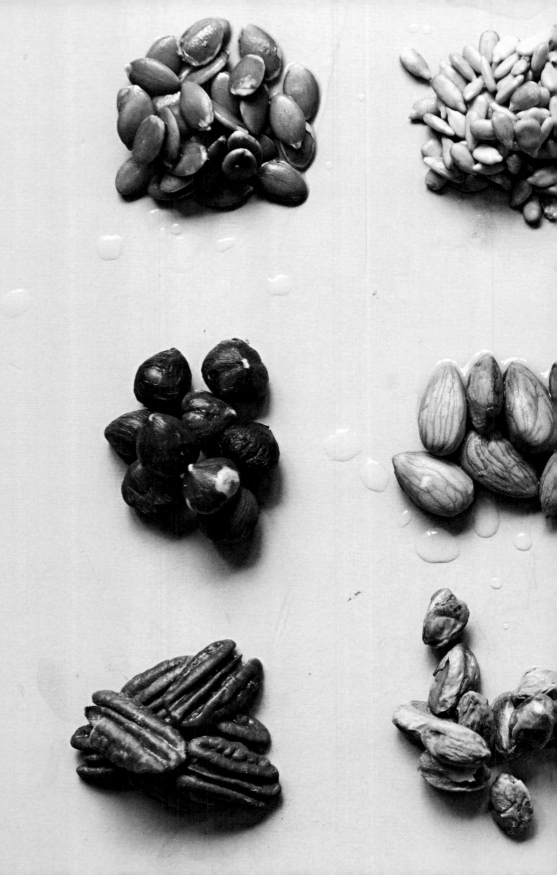

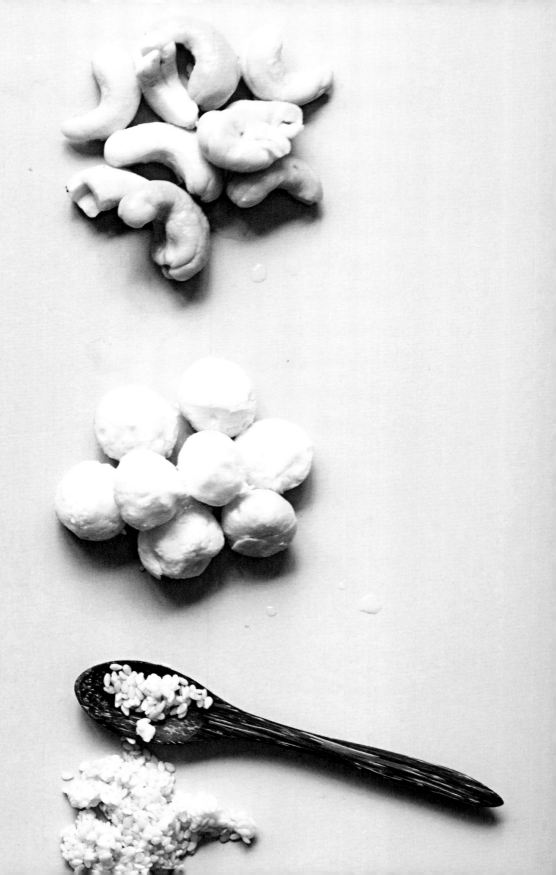

NUTS & SEEDS - A GUIDE

Nuts and seeds are nature's own smart foods. They are jam-packed with minerals, protein, antioxidants and healthy unsaturated fats. Studies have shown that the risk of cardiovascular disease, among other illnesses, may decrease in those who consume nuts regularly in moderate amounts.

In this section, I mention useful techniques to get the most from nuts and seeds when making vegan dairy products. I also detail some of my favourite types of nuts and seeds (and oats!) that I use in the book.

WHAT IS A NUT?

Botanically speaking, nuts are defined as single-seeded fruits that are hard, dry and encased in a shell. Yet, the word 'nut' also covers edible fruit stones or drupes, as well as pistachios that are actually seeds, and not forgetting peanuts that are legumes. However, what all nuts have in common is that they make delicious vegan dairy products.

SOAKING

Unpasteurized or raw nuts contain phytic acid, which means that our bodies can't absorb the minerals found in them. While enzyme inhibiting substances also found in nuts can make them difficult to digest. The answer is to soak them before use so they are easier to digest and their minerals are more accessible and can be absorbed by the body. Soaked nuts also have a milder, rounder flavour and are much softer and easier to blend or grind. In most cases, the nuts you buy from shops are pasteurized, but I would still recommend soaking them first just in case. I also suggest soaking seeds for the same reasons.

To soak nuts (and seeds), place them in a jar and cover with water – room temperature, not chilled. Put the lid on and leave to stand in the fridge overnight. The next morning, drain the nuts (and seeds) and rinse them in clean water. Use them to make vegan milk, cheese, cream or yogurt, or you can activate the nuts (see page 22) to make nut butter or flour.

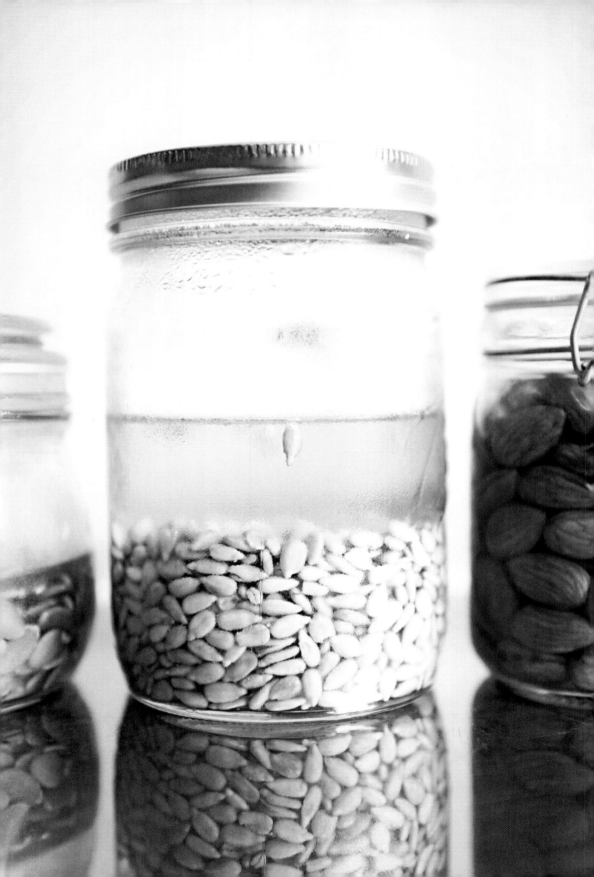

ACTIVATING

Activated or dried nuts are super delicious made into butter, ground into flour or eaten as a snack with a little sprinkling of sea salt. Activating nuts involves drying them at a low heat after soaking. Drying can take 8–12 hours in a dehydrator, but if you haven't got one, then you can dry them in a standard oven. To do this, preheat the oven to 110°C/225°F/Gas Mark ¼. Place the nuts on a baking tray (sheet) in the oven for 12–24 hours until dry and crisp. It also possible to activate or dry seeds using the same methods.

NUTRITION AND SOAKING TIMES

Here is a selection of my favourite nuts and seeds (and oats) with approximate soaking times where relevant.

Cashew nuts

The cashew nut is packed with fibre, protein and antioxidants as well as minerals such as magnesium and zinc. It's one of the most popular nuts for making vegan dairy products since it has a great creamy texture and flavour and is very easy to buy.
Soaking time: 8 hours.

Hazelnuts

The hazelnut is rich in B vitamins and vitamin E as well as minerals such as phosphorus, calcium and magnesium. Personally, I think they taste best toasted, but they're not too shabby used in chocolate milk either.
Soaking time: 8 hours.

Peanuts

The peanut is rich in protein and fat and has a high fibre content. Peanut butter is probably the most popular nut butter and it's ridiculously tasty.
Soaking time: 8 hours.

Coconut

What a super nut – well, it's actually a stone fruit! The flesh of the coconut is packed with fibre and minerals. The coconut is very versatile, the flesh is grated (shredded) into flakes, pressed to produce oil, while coconut sugar is made using the nectar from the coconut palm's flowers.
Soaking time: None.

Macadamia nuts

My personal favourite nut. I love this fatty, creamy nut, which comes from Australia. The macadamia makes excellent nut butters, cream and milk and is rich in iron, magnesium and omega-3 fats.

Soaking time: 8 hours.

Almonds

The almond is the most nutritious nut available. It contains high levels of magnesium and vitamins B and E, which are great for supporting the immune system. The almond is also rich in iron, fibre and protein. Use blanched almonds, or if they still have their skins on, rub them off the nuts after soaking.

Soaking time: 8–12 hours.

Pecan nuts

This beautiful brown nut originates from the southern parts of America and is rich in unsaturated fat and protein. Traditionally, the nut is used in desserts and ice creams, but it works perfectly in vegan milk and butter as well.

Soaking time: 4–6 hours.

Pistachio nuts

A crunchy nut with high levels of antioxidants that help maintain healthy cholesterol levels in the body. With origins in the Middle East, pistachios are pretty expensive, but are so incredibly delicious. Look for unsalted ones.

Soaking time: 6 hours.

Walnuts

The walnut is rich in omega-3 fats, vitamin E, magnesium and antioxidants. This combination of nutrients and because it actually looks like a brain are the reasons why I like to call it the 'brain nut' – it contains a whole lot of what our brains actually need!

Soaking time: 8 hours.

Hemp seeds

Hemp seeds are a favourite. They are so easy to use as they don't need pre-soaking (especially the hulled or shelled variety) and can be added to all kinds of recipes. Hemp seeds are rich in protein, fibre and omega-3 fats.

Soaking time: None.

Pumpkin seeds
Pumpkin seeds are mainly rich in minerals and vitamin E. They are great to use in vegan dairy products and can be added to a variety of dishes.
Soaking time: 8 hours.

Sesame seeds
Sesame seeds are calcium-rich and are traditionally used whole in Asian cooking, but the tiny seeds are also turned into spreads, butters and pastes in Arabic and North African dishes.
Soaking time: 8 hours.

Sunflower seeds
Sunflower seeds are super tasty just as they are or when toasted and can be used in salads, muesli and breads. They're a favourite of mine in vegan dairy products, since the seeds are fairly cheap and easy to use. Sunflower seeds are rich in B vitamins and minerals, particularly magnesium.
Soaking time: 2 hours.

Oats
Although not a nut or a seed, oats are a really good friend of your heart – they contain beta glucans, a type of dietary fibre that can lower cholesterol levels in the body. Beta glucans have a jelly-like consistency when soaked, so when making oat milk it's important to use the right amount or the milk can have a slimy consistency. Oats are also a fantastic source of protein. And best of all? Oats are super cheap. Making oat-based milk, porridge, muesli and energy bars is not just healthy for you, but is good economically too.
Soaking time: None.

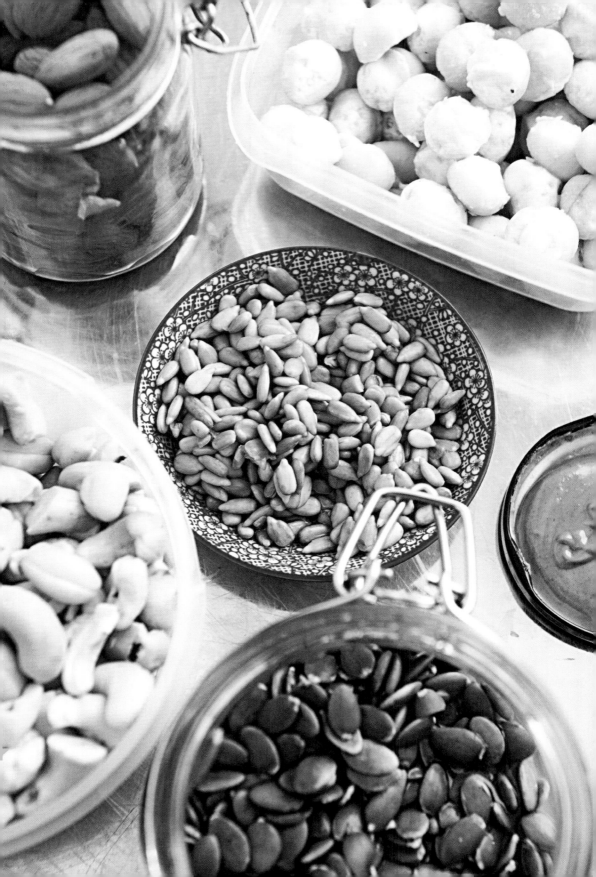

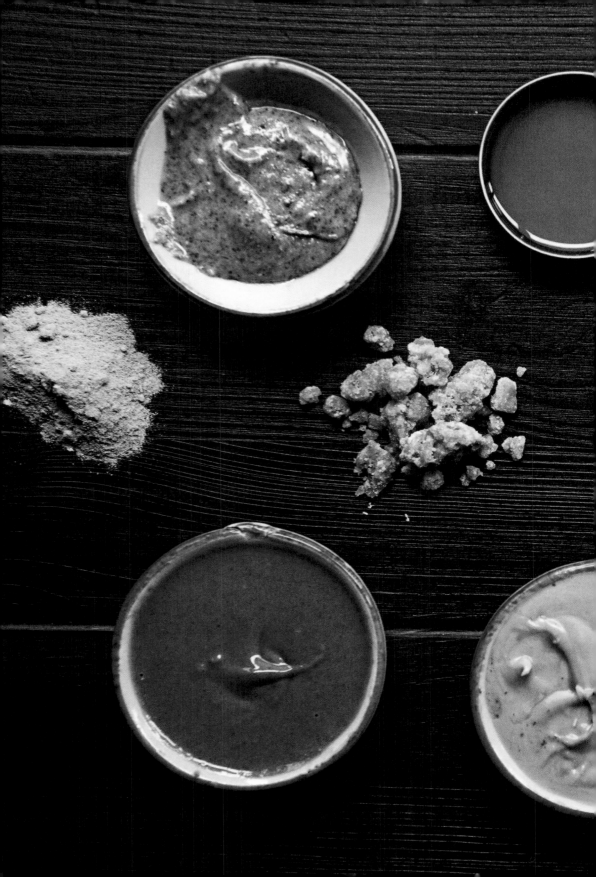

Nut & seed butters

Nut and seed butters are so rewarding to make for a number of reasons: they're simple, super tasty, and fun to try out different types and flavour combinations. There are a range of butters in this chapter, from the very basic and simple to those flavoured with interesting spices – both sweet and savoury. This chapter also includes Almond Butter (see page 29) for those who want an alternative to more traditional dairy butter to spread on bread or to use in baking and cooking.

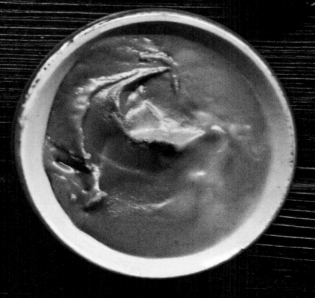

กำลังทรพี กำลังเพ็ชหึง

ล้ว ป.ทองหลางหนาม ป.ทองหลางใบมล

ร.เลี่ย ชุมพร

ร.กะทุงหมาบ้า ร.กะทุงลาย

รากกะท้อน ร.กะทุกลด

รากรกฟ้า ร.ราชมานพ

Almond butter

This butter is really creamy with a nutty flavour. It's nice spread on toast and is good for baking, cooking and in Asian dressings.

MAKES ABOUT 200G/7OZ/1½ CUPS

200g/7oz/1½ cups almonds
a little sea salt

Add the almonds and salt to a food processor and blend on the highest speed for 20–30 minutes until smooth. Pause every now and again to scrape down the contents from the sides of the mixer bowl.

Spoon into a clean jar with a tight-fitting lid and store in the fridge. The butter will keep for about 3 weeks.

Almond and coconut butter with chia seeds

Use this butter in smoothies, desserts, ice cream and for baking.

MAKES ABOUT 400G/14OZ/HEAPED 3½ CUPS

300g/10½ oz/2¼ cups almonds
100g/3½ oz/1⅓ cups desiccated (shredded) coconut
1 tbsp chia seeds

Preheat the oven to 180°C/350°F/Gas Mark 4. Place the almonds on a baking tray (sheet) and toast for 15 minutes until golden. Toast the coconut in a dry pan on a medium heat until coloured, 2–3 minutes. Leave to cool.

Add the almonds and coconut to a food processor and blend on the highest speed for 15–20 minutes until smooth. Pause every now and again to scrape down the contents from the sides of the mixer bowl. Stir in the chia seeds.

Spoon into a clean jar with a tight-fitting lid and store in the fridge. The butter will keep for about 3 weeks.

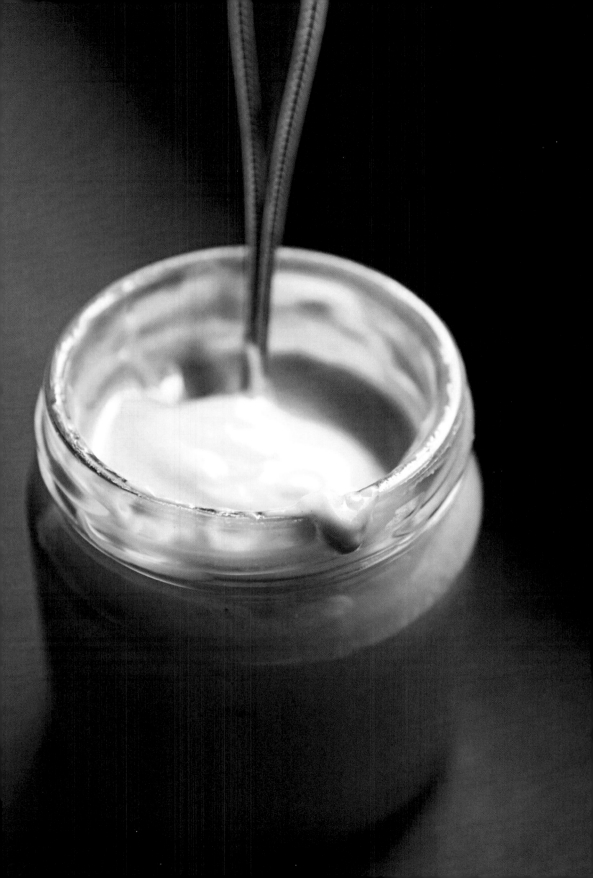

Cashew butter

Cashew butter is delicious in salad dressings, as a sandwich topper and for baking. The cashew nut is naturally sweet and creamy, which makes it good in nut creams too.

MAKES ABOUT 200G/7OZ/1½ CUPS

200g/7oz/heaped 1½ cups cashew nuts
1 tsp sea salt

Add the cashews and salt to a food processor and blend on the highest speed for 20–30 minutes until smooth. Pause every now and again to scrape down the contents from the sides of the mixer bowl.

Spoon into a clean jar with a tight-fitting lid and store in the fridge. The butter will keep for about 3 weeks.

Coconut butter

Coconut butter is quick to make, it only takes a minute or two in a food processor. I use the butter for smoothies and dressings.

MAKES ABOUT 150G/5½ OZ/2 CUPS

150g/5½ oz/2 cups desiccated (shredded) coconut
1 tbsp coconut oil, melted
½ tsp vanilla powder
a pinch of sea salt

Add all the ingredients to a food processor and blend on the highest speed for 1 minute or until smooth.

Spoon into a clean jar with a tight-fitting lid and store in the fridge. The butter will keep for about 3 weeks.

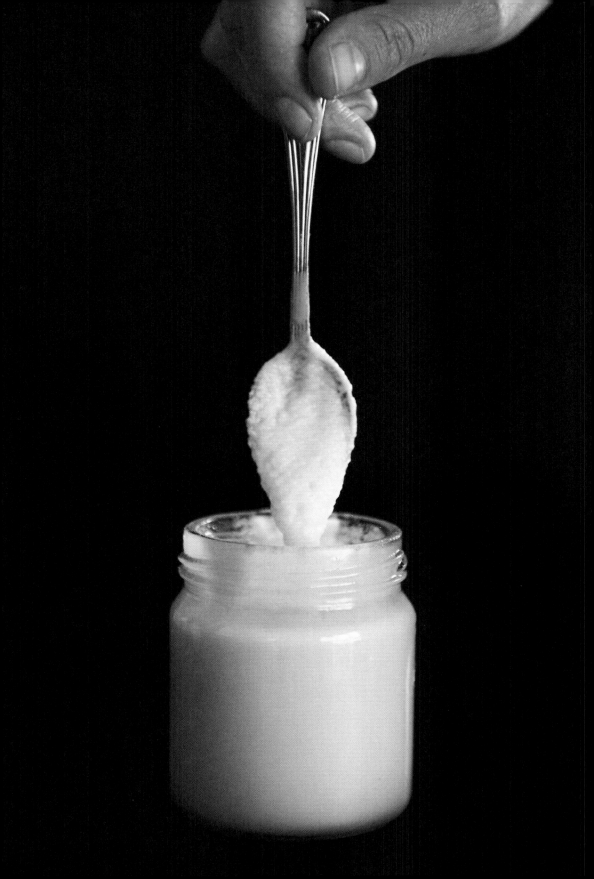

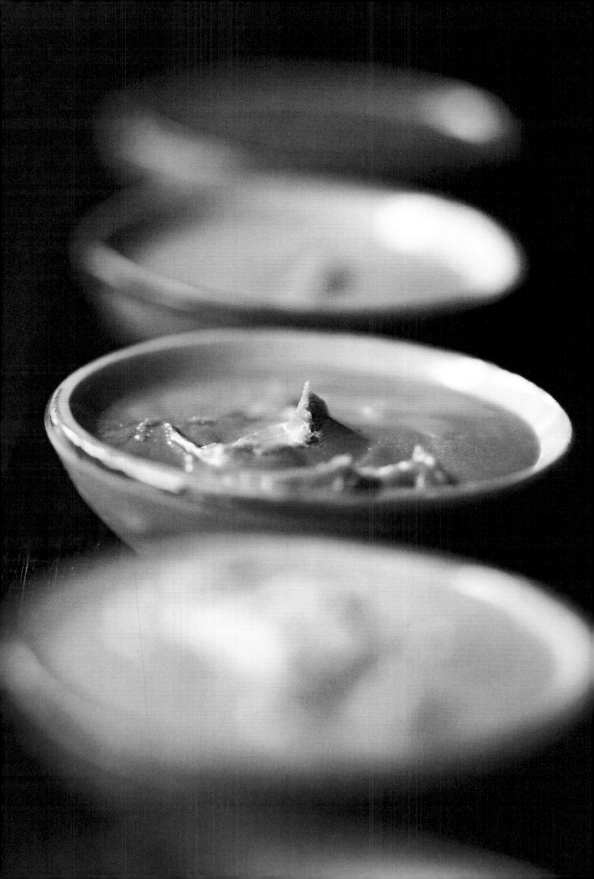

Pecan nut butter

With a touch of cinnamon spice, this butter is good in desserts or added to a breakfast porridge bowl.

MAKES ABOUT 350G/12OZ/3 CUPS

350g/12oz/3 cups pecan nuts
a pinch of sea salt
½ tsp ground cinnamon

Toast the pecans in a dry pan on a medium heat for 5 minutes or until lightly coloured. Remove from the heat.

Add all the ingredients to a food processor and blend on the highest speed for a few minutes until smooth. Pause every now and again to scrape down the contents from the sides of the mixer bowl.

Spoon into a clean jar with a tight-fitting lid and store in the fridge. The butter will keep for about 2–3 weeks.

Peanut
butter

The nut butter of nut butters! There's no reason to buy ready-made since it's so easy to make it yourself. This butter is good on bread with marmalade, in smoothies or in ice cream.

MAKES ABOUT 400G/14OZ/4 CUPS

400g/14oz/4 cups unsalted peanuts
2 tsp maple syrup
a little sea salt
2 tbsp coconut oil, melted (you may not need this)

Preheat the oven to 175°C/350°F/Gas Mark 4.

Roast the peanuts in a baking dish for 6 minutes, shaking the nuts halfway through, until lightly coloured. Leave to cool.

Add all the ingredients to a food processor and blend on the highest speed for 2–3 minutes until smooth. Add the oil if the mixture is difficult to work. Pause every now and again to scrape down the contents from the sides of the mixer bowl.

Spoon into a clean jar with a tight-fitting lid and store in the fridge. The butter will keep for about 4 weeks.

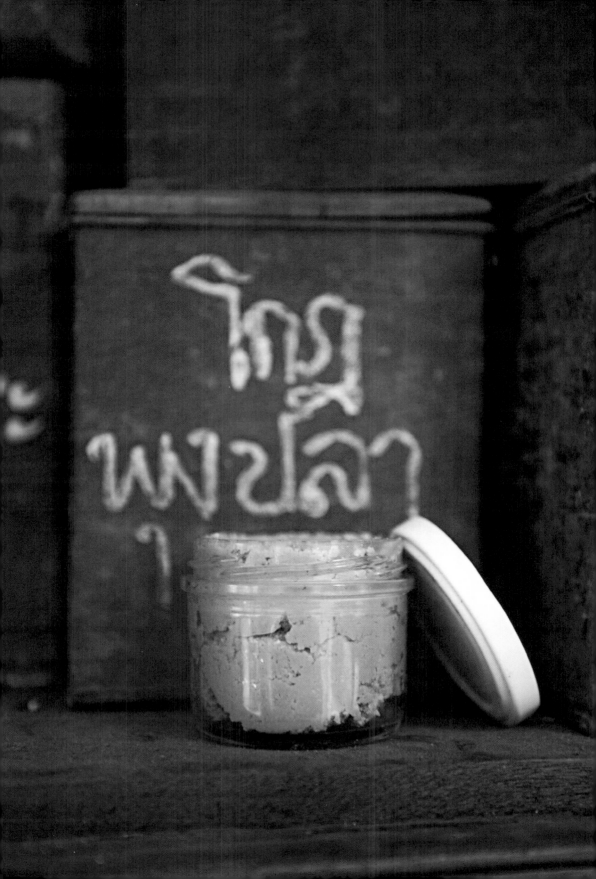

Pistachio butter

Pistachio butter is super nice with sweet sauces and jam. I like to spread it onto pancakes and top them with coconut syrup and coconut flakes.

MAKES ABOUT 280G/10OZ/2¼ CUPS

280g/10oz/2¼ cups shelled unsalted pistachio nuts

1 tsp sea salt

1 tbsp maple syrup

½ tsp ground cinnamon

Add the nuts to a food processor and blend on the highest speed for 10 minutes, then add the rest of the ingredients and blend for a further 10 minutes until smooth. Pause every now and again to scrape down the contents from the sides of the mixer bowl.

Spoon into a clean jar with a tight-fitting lid and store in the fridge. The butter will keep for about 3 weeks.

Sesame butter and Tahini

Sesame butter is one of my favourite recipes since it has so many uses. Likewise, sesame seed paste or tahini, which is an essential ingredient in my kitchen. Both add creaminess and flavour, whether they're added to bread, hummus or dressings.

MAKES ABOUT 200G/7OZ/1½ CUPS

200g/7oz/1½ cups sesame seeds, toasted or untoasted

2–6 tbsp olive oil

a pinch of sea salt

Add the sesame seeds, the smaller quantity of oil and the salt to a food processor and blend on the highest speed for 5 minutes or until smooth. Add more oil if the mixture is difficult to work.

Spoon into a clean jar with a tight-fitting lid and store in the fridge. The butter will keep for about 3 weeks.

– To make tahini, add more oil for a looser consistency.

TIP

Use black sesame seeds for an exciting colour variation.

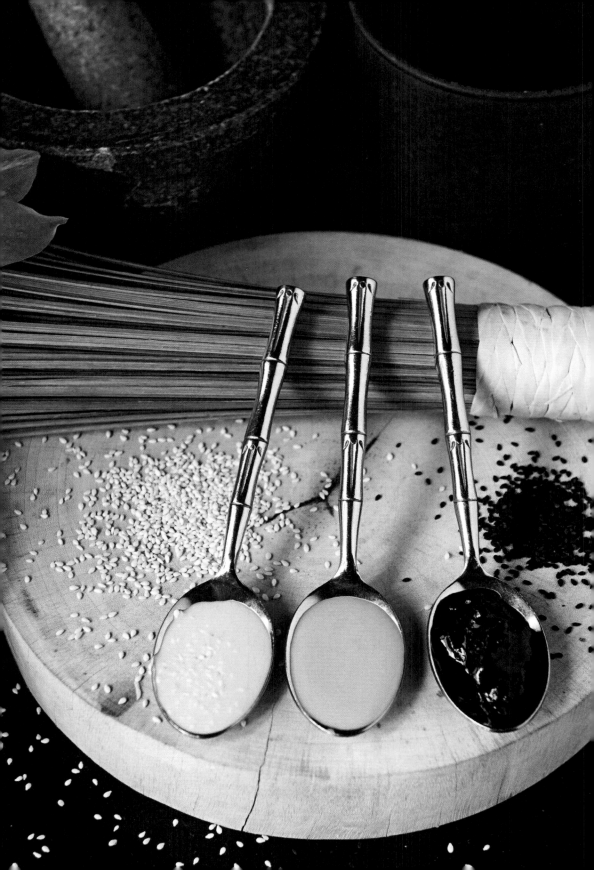

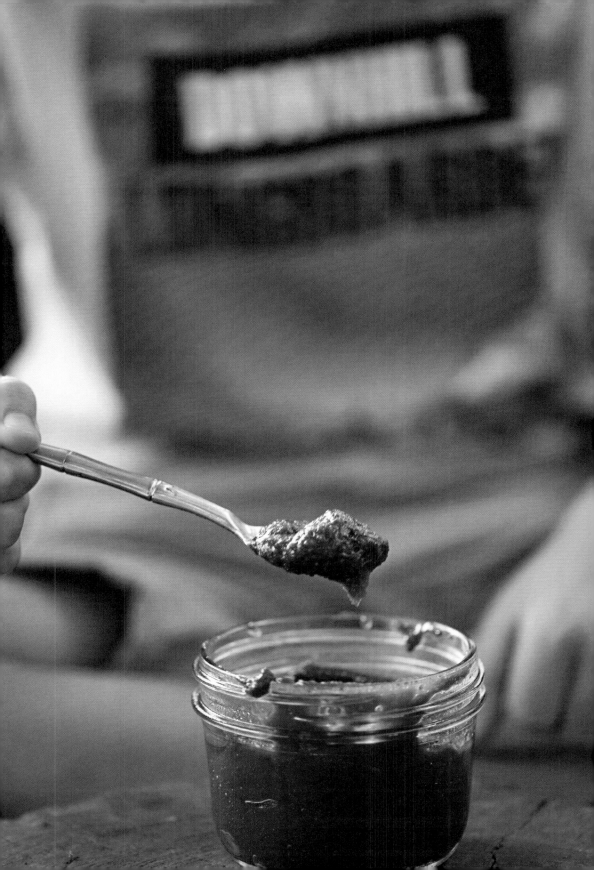

Chocolate and hazelnut butter

Nutella or chocolate spread without palm oil and additives, how does that sound? After you've made your first batch of this you won't want to buy shop-bought versions again. This nutty, creamy, chocolatey butter works well in desserts, sauces, smoothies and just straight up as it comes.

MAKES ABOUT 200G/7OZ/1½ CUPS

200g/7oz/1½ cups hazelnuts
1 tbsp coconut oil, melted
2 tbsp cacao powder
3 tbsp maple syrup
½ tsp sea salt

Preheat the oven to 180°C/350°F/Gas Mark 4.

Mix together the nuts, oil, cacao powder, syrup and salt in a bowl. Spread out the mixture on a baking tray (sheet) lined with baking (parchment) paper and roast for 15 minutes or until the nuts are golden. Leave to cool.

Add the mixture to a food processor and blend on the highest speed for a few minutes until smooth. Pause every now and again to scrape down the contents from the sides of the mixer bowl.

Spoon into a clean jar with a tight-fitting lid and store in the fridge. The butter will keep for about 3 weeks.

Pumpkin seed butter

The lovely colour from the pumpkin seeds means this butter is the most beautiful of the bunch – it's also delicious and nutritious. I use it when I want to make a quick pumpkin seed milk (1 tbsp butter added to 400ml/14fl oz/1¾ cups water) as well as in dressings and sauces.

MAKES ABOUT 350G/12OZ/2½ CUPS

350g/12oz/2½ cups pumpkin seeds

a little sea salt

2–3 tbsp coconut oil, melted (you may not need this)

Add the seeds and salt to a food processor and blend on the highest speed for a few minutes until smooth. Pause every now and again to scrape down the contents from the sides of the mixer bowl. Add the coconut oil towards the end if the butter is very stiff, adding the small amount first.

Spoon into a clean jar with a tight-fitting lid and store in the fridge. The butter will keep for about 3 weeks.

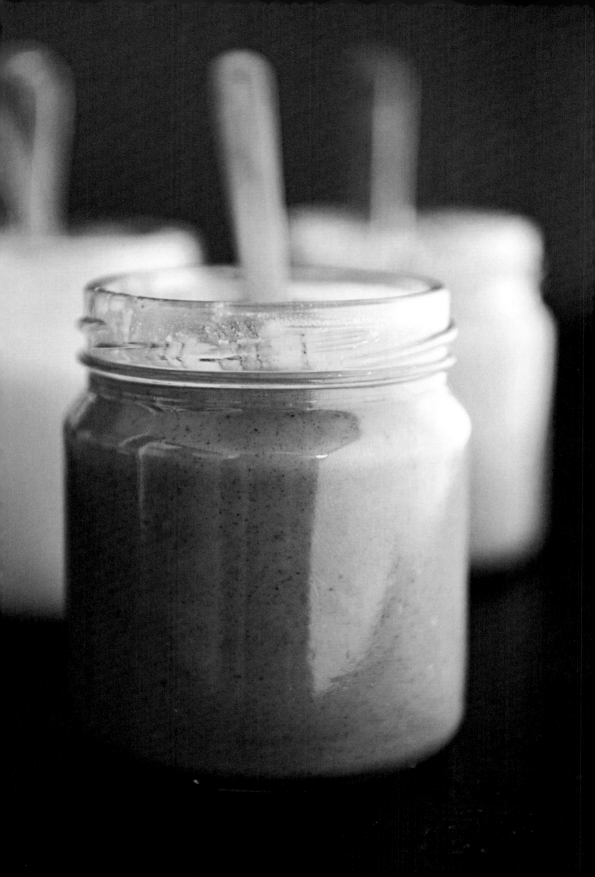

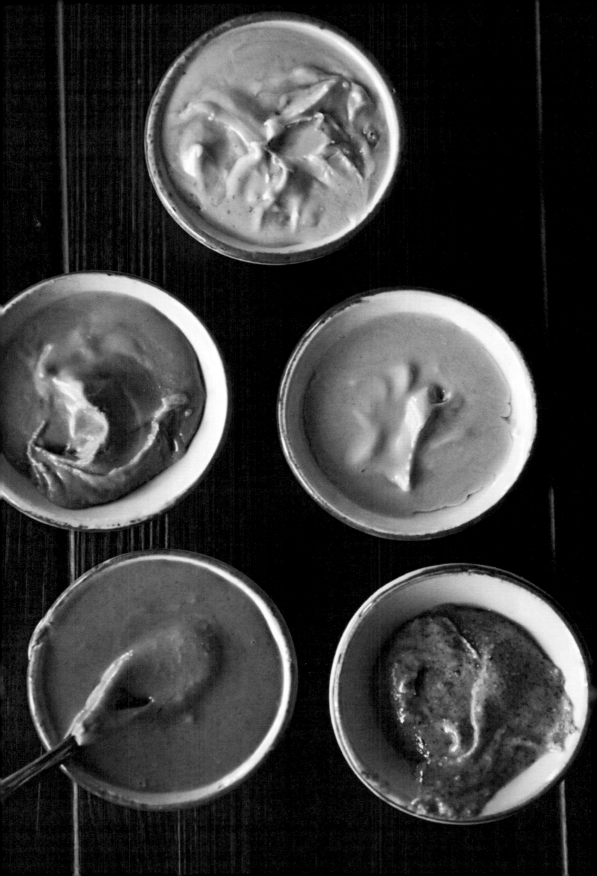

Spicy pumpkin seed butter

Pumpkin seeds, cinnamon and ginger are flavours that marry well. Try adding a spoonful of this to your gingerbread dough or other favourite biscuit mixture. It's also good in smoothies.

MAKES ABOUT 350G/12OZ/2½ CUPS

350g/12oz/2½ cups pumpkin seeds, toasted
1 tbsp coconut syrup
⅓ tsp ground cinnamon
⅓ tsp ginger, grated fresh or dried

Add the seeds, coconut syrup and spices to a food processor and blend on the highest speed for 10 minutes until smooth. Pause every now and again to scrape down the contents from the sides of the mixer bowl.

Spoon into a clean jar with a tight-fitting lid and store in the fridge. The butter will keep for about 3 weeks.

Clockwise from top: Peacan Nut Butter, Cashew Butter, Vanilla and Pecan Butter, Spicy Pumpkin Seed Butter, Cashew and Walnut Butter.

Lemon and pistachio butter

This citrusy butter works perfectly as a light pesto, or stirred into sauces and dressings, and as a dip for crudités.

MAKES ABOUT 225G/8OZ/1¾ CUPS

225g/8oz/1¾ cups shelled unsalted pistachio nuts

2 tbsp lemon juice

1 tsp finely grated lemon zest

2 tbsp olive oil

Add the nuts to a food processor and blend on the highest speed for a few minutes until smooth. Pause every now and again to scrape down the contents from the sides of the mixer bowl. When the nuts are smooth, add the rest of the ingredients and blend briefly again.

Spoon into a clean jar with a tight-fitting lid and store in the fridge. The butter will keep for about 3 weeks.

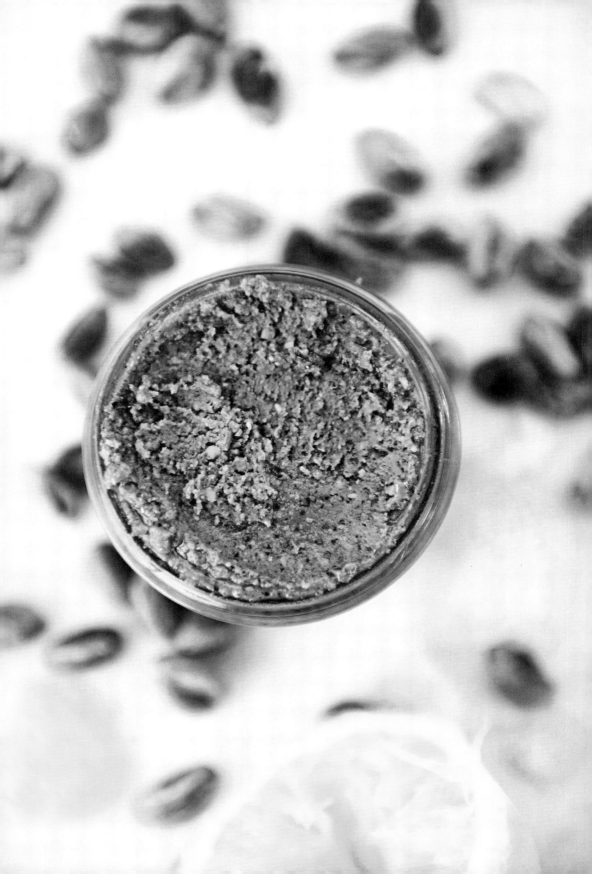

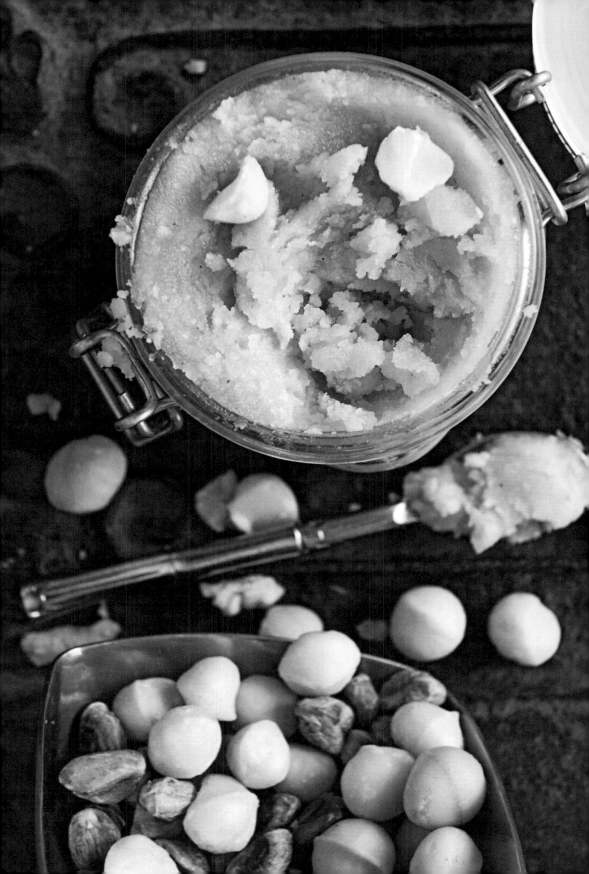

Toasted macadamia butter

Macadamia nuts make a luxurious, world-class butter. The nuts have a creamy texture that makes the butter... extra creamy. It's delicious with everything, but is particularly good in rich chocolate desserts.

MAKES ABOUT 350G/12OZ/ 3 CUPS

350g/12oz/scant 3 cups macadamia nuts
2 tbsp maple syrup
4 tbsp coconut oil, melted
a pinch of sea salt
½ tsp ground cinnamon

Preheat the oven to 180°C/350°F/Gas Mark 4.

Mix together the nuts, syrup, oil, salt and cinnamon in a bowl. Spread out the mixture onto a baking tray (sheet) lined with baking (parchment) paper and roast for 15 minutes or until the nuts have turned golden. Leave to cool.

Add the mixture to a food processor and blend on the highest speed for 20 minutes until smooth. Pause every now and again to scrapedown the contents from the sides of the mixer bowl.

Spoon into a clean jar with a tight-fitting lid and store in the fridge. The butter will keep for about 3 weeks.

Vanilla and pecan butter

Pecan nuts and vanilla are a successful combo. This butter works well in ice cream or baking such as in a filling for buns or icing for a cake.

MAKES ABOUT 280G/ 10OZ/2¼ CUPS

280g/10oz/2¼ cups pecan nuts
2 tbsp coconut oil, melted
1 tsp vanilla powder

Preheat the oven to 180°C/350°F/Gas Mark 4.

Place the nuts on a baking tray (sheet) lined with baking (parchment) paper and roast for 5 minutes or until the nuts have turned light golden. Leave to cool.

Add all the ingredients to a food processor and blend on the highest speed for 15–30 minutes until smooth. Pause every now and again to scrape down the contents from the sides of the mixer bowl.

Spoon into a clean jar with a tight-fitting lid and store in the fridge. The butter will keep for about 3 weeks.

Clockwise from top: Spicy Pumpkin Seed Butter, Pecan Nut Butter, Vanilla and Pecan Butter, Cashew and Walnut Butter, Cashew Butter.

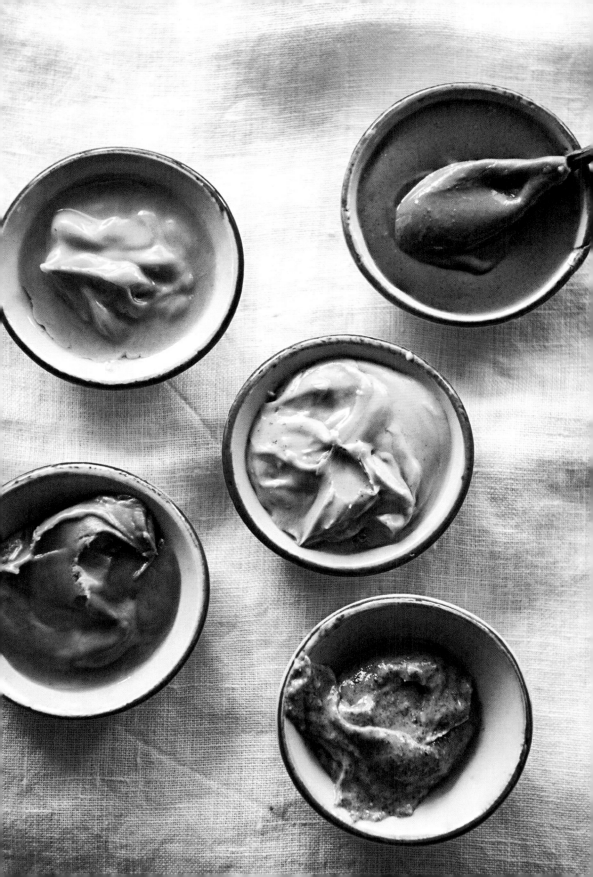

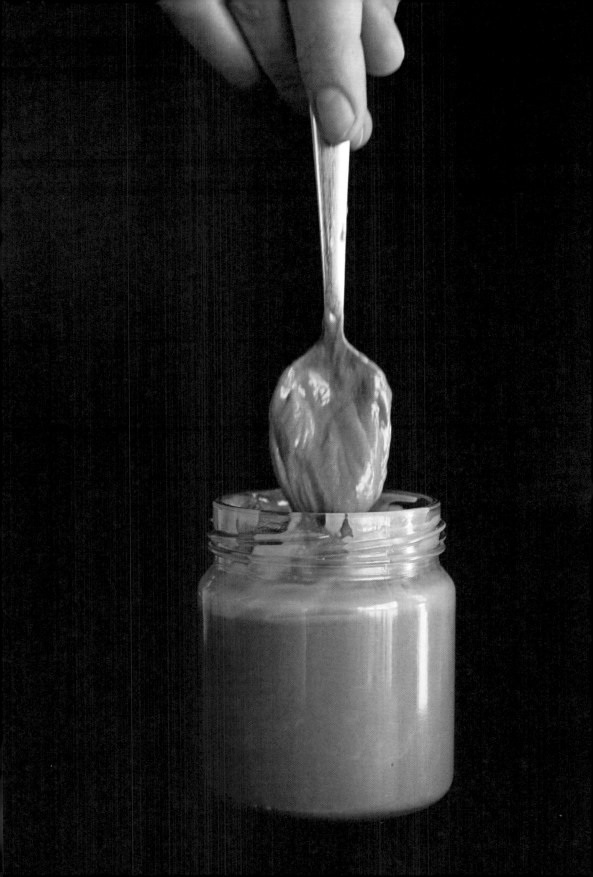

Cashew and walnut butter

This combination of roasted nuts is really delicious. The maple syrup and coconut counterbalance the slightly bitter taste of the walnuts.

MAKES ABOUT 225G/ 8OZ/HEAPED 1½ CUPS

140g/5oz/heaped
  1 cup cashew nuts
70g/2½ oz/½ cup
  walnuts
1 tbsp desiccated
  (shredded) coconut
2 tbsp maple syrup

Preheat the oven to 180°C/350°F/Gas Mark 4.

Place the cashews, walnuts and coconut on a baking tray (sheet) lined with baking (parchment) paper and roast for 5 minutes or until the nuts have turned light golden. Leave to cool.

Add all the ingredients to a food processor and blend on the highest speed for 15–30 minutes until smooth. Pause every now and again to scrape down the contents from the sides of the mixer bowl.

Spoon into a clean jar with a tight-fitting lid and store in the fridge. The butter will keep for about 3 weeks.

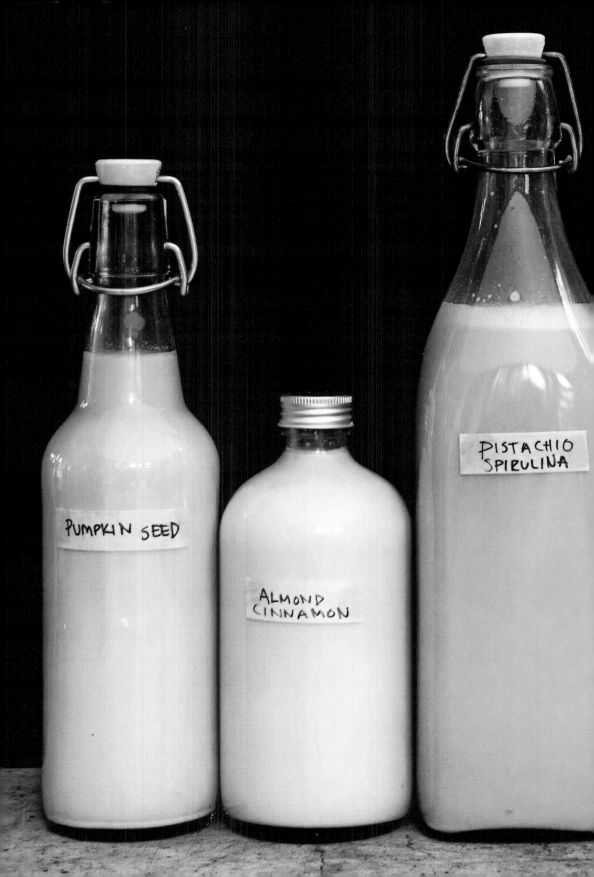

Vegan milks

Nut, seed and grain milks can vary a lot in flavour depending on which ingredients you use. Here, you can be creative with flavourings, but when it comes to the ratio of liquid to nuts, seeds or grains, you have to be careful since if the balance is out it can affect the consistency of the milk. Oats, for example, due to their starch content can become a bit slimy if you use more than what is stated in the recipe.

Most vegan milks will keep for 2–4 days in the fridge. If you don't want to use hot water you can use cold instead. I tend to use hot because it draws out the flavours a bit more and also softens the texture of the nuts and seeds. Always save the pulp that's left over – the bit that's in the nut bag after draining – it can be used for baking. If you own a dehydrator, try drying the pulp into flour.

HEMP SEED

MACADAMIA
STRAWBERRY

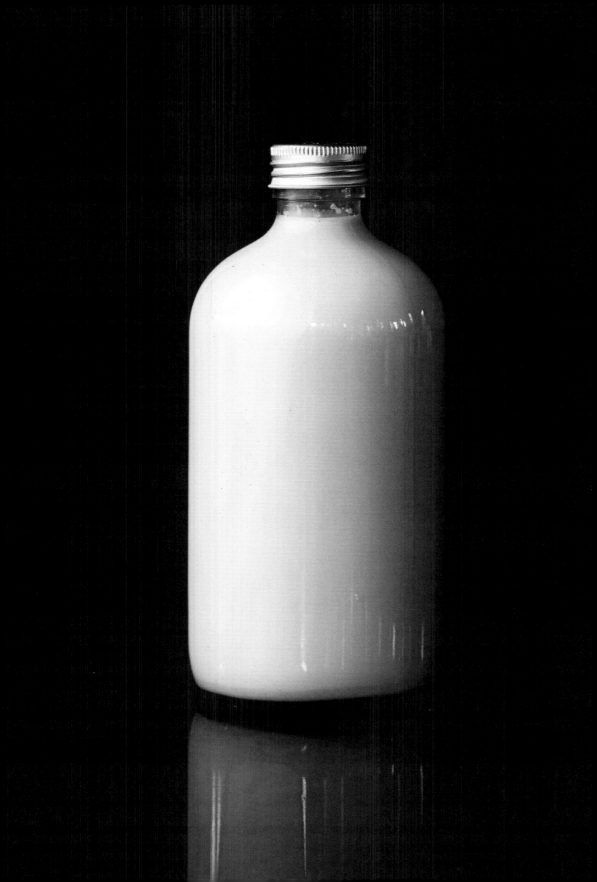

Almond milk

The simplest transition from regular dairy to vegan dairy is to make almond milk. Almonds are so easy to get hold of and are a very familiar nut to most of us. Almond milk is nice in coffee, smoothies and poured over muesli or granola.

MAKES ABOUT 1 LITRE/1¾ PINTS/GENEROUS 4 CUPS

225g/8oz/scant 1¾ cups almonds, soaked, drained and rinsed (see page 20)

½ tsp vanilla powder

½ tsp ground cinnamon

a pinch of sea salt

3 medjool dates, pitted and chopped

1 litre/1¼ pints/generous 4 cups hot water

Put all the ingredients in a blender and blend for 2–3 minutes until smooth. Pour the contents into a nut bag, placed in a bowl. Twist the bag to squeeze the liquid into the bowl and leave to cool.

Pour the milk into a clean bottle with a tight-fitting lid. Place in the fridge and leave to stand for a couple of hours or overnight before using. Store in the fridge and use within 2 days.

Quick almond milk

A perfect recipe for those who haven't got the time or have forgotten to pre-soak the almonds.

MAKES ABOUT 1 LITRE/1¾ PINTS/GENEROUS 4 CUPS

1 litre/1¾ pints/generous 4 cups water
3 tbsp Almond Butter (see page 29)
a pinch of sea salt

Put all the ingredients in a blender and blend for 1 minute or until smooth.

Pour the milk into a clean bottle with a tight-fitting lid. Store in the fridge and use within 2 days.

TIP
Almond butter is good to have to hand
if you want to make a quick nut milk.

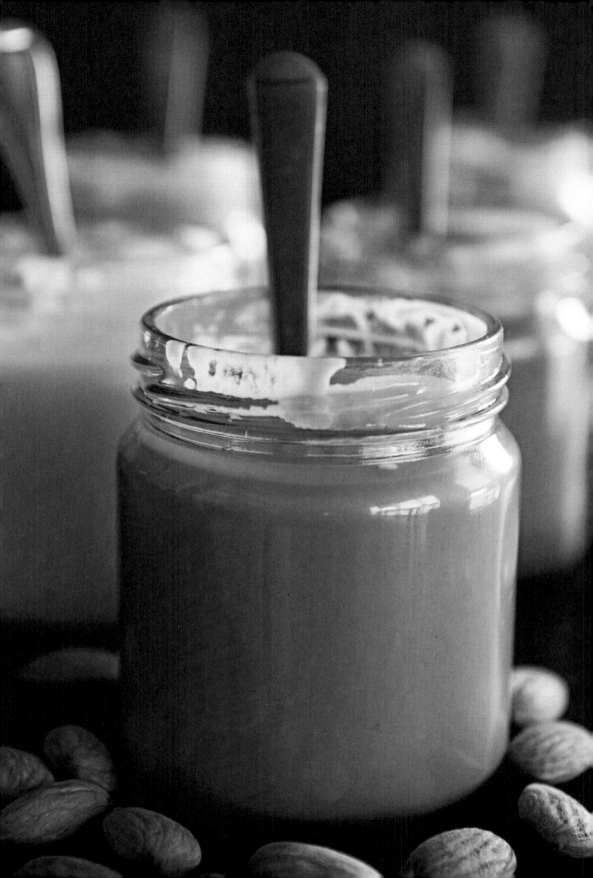

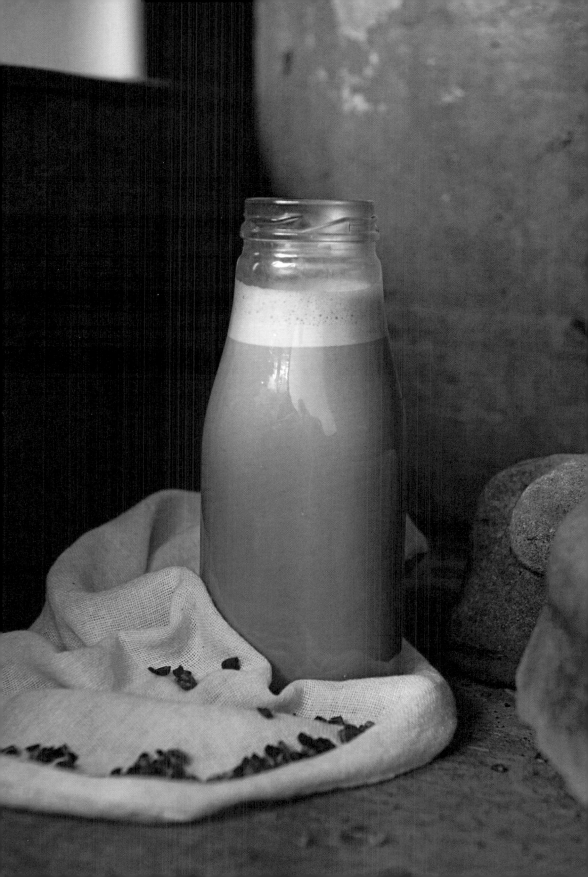

Chocolate and hazelnut milk

This chocolate milk makes a delicious treat and is highly nutritious. Share it, either warm or cold, with friends.

MAKES ABOUT 1 LITRE/1¾ PINTS/GENEROUS 4 CUPS

1 vanilla pod
185g/6½oz/scant 1½ cups hazelnuts
1 litre/1¾ pints/generous 4 cups hot water
½ tsp sea salt
2 tbsp maple syrup
2 tbsp cacao powder

Soak the vanilla pod and nuts in a jug of water for about 8 hours. Strain and rinse thoroughly. Cut the vanilla pod lengthways and scrape out the seeds.

Add the nuts, vanilla seeds, water, salt, syrup and cacao powder to a blender and blend for 2 minutes or until the hazelnuts are very finely chopped. Pour the contents into a nut bag, placed in a bowl. Twist the bag to squeeze the liquid into the bowl and leave to cool.

Pour the milk into a clean bottle with a tight-fitting lid. Place in the fridge and leave to stand for a couple of hours or overnight before using. Store in the fridge and use within 2 days. It can also be enjoyed hot!

Sesame milk

Sesame milk with dates reminds me of Middle Eastern-style food. Using hot water allows the flavours to come through more, but isn't essential. Serve warm or cold as a drink or with porridge or in smoothies.

MAKES ABOUT 1 LITRE/1¾ PINTS/GENEROUS 4 CUPS

1 vanilla pod
185g/6½ oz/scant 1½ cups sesame seeds, soaked, drained and rinsed (see page 20)
3 medjool dates, pitted and chopped
1 litre/1¾ pints/generous 4 cups hot water

Cut the vanilla pod lengthways and scrape out the seeds. Put the vanilla seeds, sesame seeds, dates and water in a blender and blend for 2–3 minutes until smooth. Pour the contents into a nut bag, placed in a bowl. Twist the bag to squeeze the liquid into the bowl and leave to cool.

Pour the milk into a clean bottle with a tight-fitting lid. Place in the fridge and leave to stand for a couple of hours or overnight before using. Store in the fridge and use within 2 days.

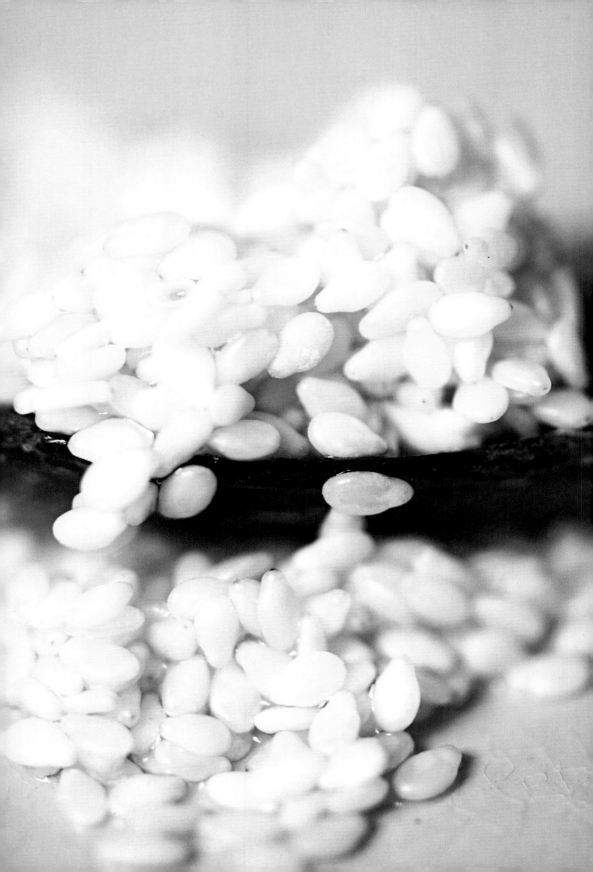

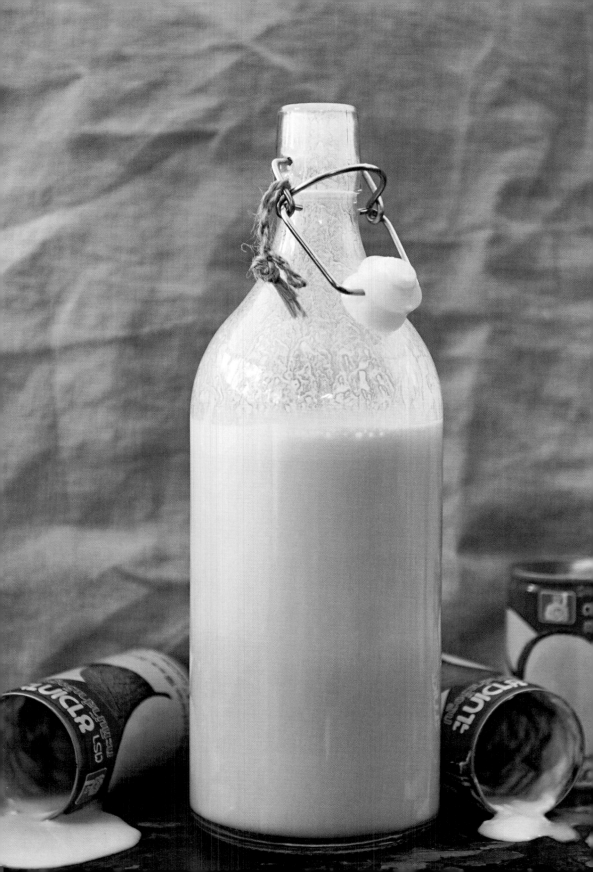

Coconut milk

You can drink canned coconut milk, but I think it has a very intense flavour that is better suited to stews or when making yogurt. This recipe makes a nice and fresh-tasting coconut drink. It's also amazing in smoothies.

MAKES ABOUT 1 LITRE/1¾ PINTS/GENEROUS 4 CUPS

300g/10½ oz/4 cups desiccated (shredded) coconut
1 litre/1¾ pints/generous 4 cups hot water

Put the coconut and water in a blender and blend for 5 minutes until smooth. Pour the contents into a nut bag, placed in a bowl. Twist the bag to squeeze the liquid into the bowl and leave to cool.

Pour the milk into a clean bottle with a tight-fitting lid. Place in the fridge and leave to stand for a couple of hours or overnight before using. Store in the fridge and use within 2 days.

Cashew milk

Cashew milk is delicious. It can be used in coffee, ice cream, yogurt and stews.

MAKES ABOUT 1 LITRE/1¾ PINTS/GENEROUS 4 CUPS

185g/6½ oz/1½ cups cashew nuts, soaked, drained
and rinsed (see page 20)
1 litre/1¾ pints/generous 4 cups hot water
1 tbsp maple syrup
a pinch of sea salt

Put all the ingredients in a blender and blend for 2–3 minutes until smooth. Pour the contents into a nut bag, placed in a bowl. Twist the bag to squeeze the liquid into the bowl and leave to cool.

Pour the milk into a clean bottle with a tight-fitting lid. Place in the fridge and leave to stand for a couple of hours or overnight before using. Store in the fridge and use within 2 days.

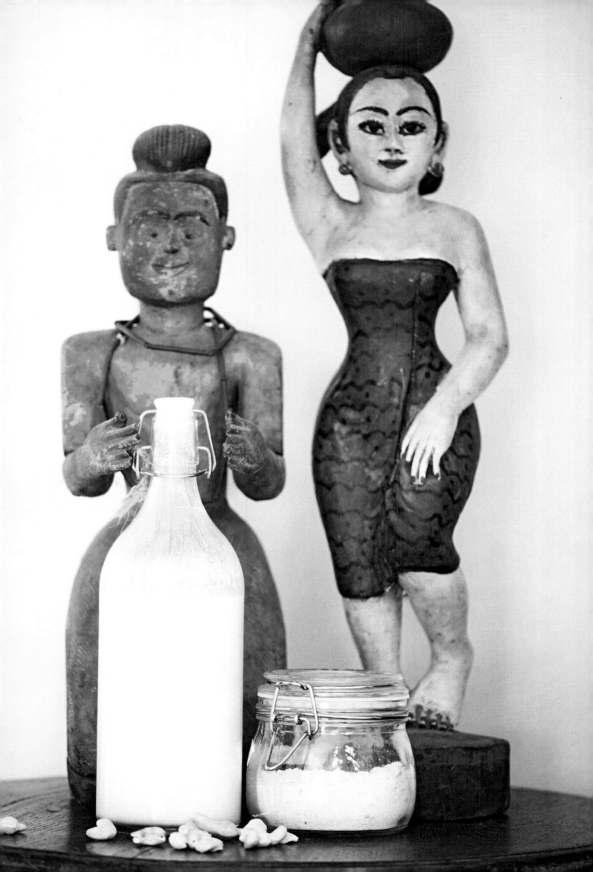

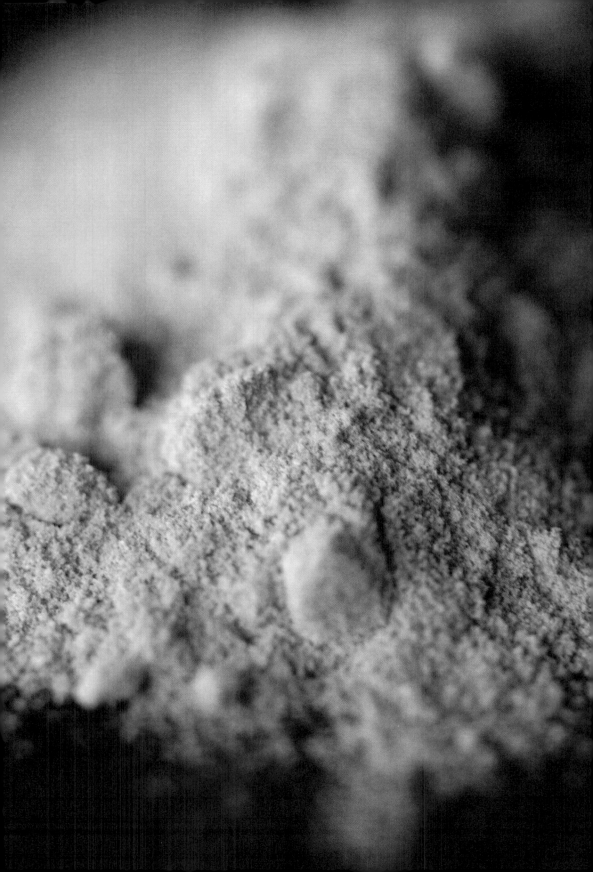

Quick cashew milk

This is a quick recipe for cashew milk if you forget to soak the nuts.

MAKES ABOUT 1 LITRE/1¾ PINTS/GENEROUS 4 CUPS

185g/6½ oz/1½ cups cashew nuts
1 litre/1¾ pints/generous 4 cups water
¼ tsp vanilla powder
a pinch of sea salt

Add the cashew nuts to a food processor and pulse to a smooth flour. Don't pulse the nuts for too long or you'll end up with butter.

Add 115g/4oz/heaped 1 cup of the cashew flour, the water, vanilla and salt to a food processor and blend on the highest speed for 1 minute or until smooth.

Pour the milk into a clean bottle with a tight-fitting lid. Store in the fridge and use within 2 days.

TIP

If you don't want to make milk from the cashew flour straight away (or you have any leftovers), transfer it to a clean jar with a tight-fitting lid. It will keep in the fridge for 3–4 days.

Oat milk

Homemade oat milk is the absolute best alternative for those who usually buy ready-made oat milk, since it's a lot cheaper and tastier. This milk is great for oat porridge or in a smoothie.

MAKES ABOUT 1 LITRE/1¾ PINTS/GENEROUS 4 CUPS

1.2 litres/2 pints/5 cups water
115g/4oz/heaped ¾ cup porridge oats (rolled oats)
a little sea salt
½ tsp vanilla powder
a pinch of ground cinnamon

Put all the ingredients in a blender and blend for 1 minute or until smooth. Pour the contents into a nut bag, placed in a bowl. Twist the bag to squeeze the liquid into the bowl.

Pour the milk into a clean bottle with a tight-fitting lid. Store in the fridge and use within 3 days.

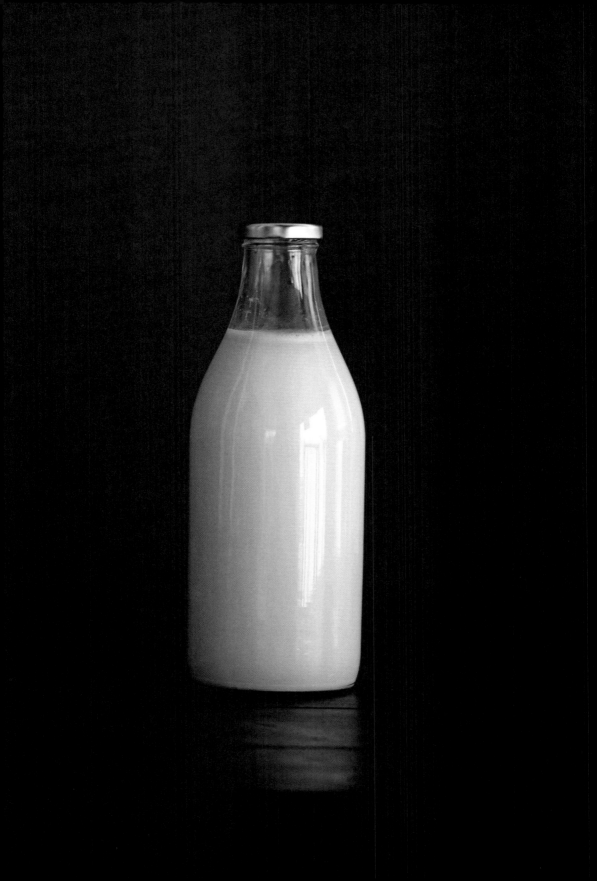

Pecan nut milk

A nutty, cinnamon-spiced milk that is good with bircher muesli, porridge or chia puddings.

MAKES ABOUT 1 LITRE/1¾ PINTS/GENEROUS 4 CUPS

175g/6oz/1½ cups pecan nuts, soaked, drained and rinsed (see page 20)

1 litre/1¾ pints/generous 4 cups hot water

5 medjool dates, pitted and chopped

2 tsp ground cinnamon

a pinch of sea salt

Put all the ingredients in a blender and blend for 2–3 minutes until smooth. Pour the contents into a nut bag, placed in a bowl. Twist the bag to squeeze the liquid into the bowl and leave to cool.

Pour the milk into a clean bottle with a tight-fitting lid. Place in the fridge and leave to stand for a couple of hours or overnight before using. Store in the fridge and use within 2 days.

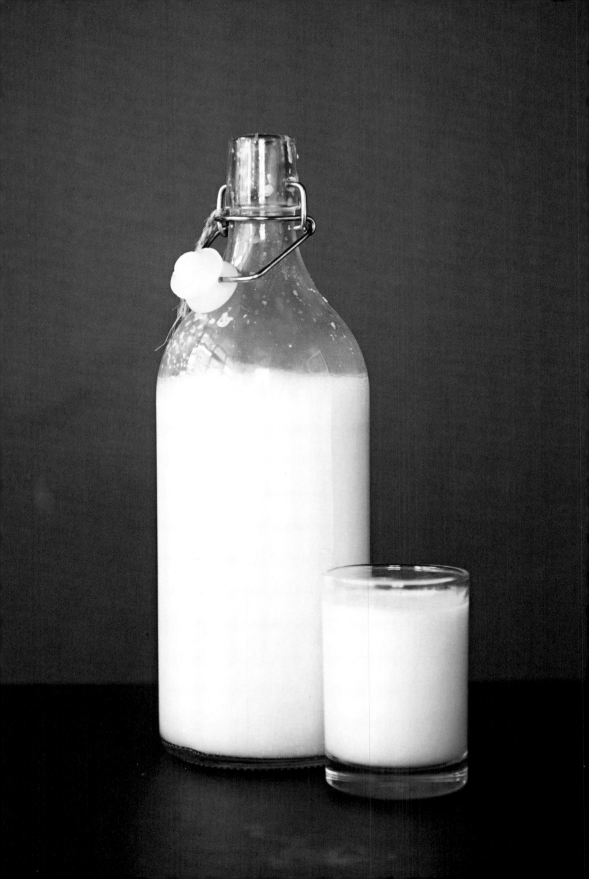

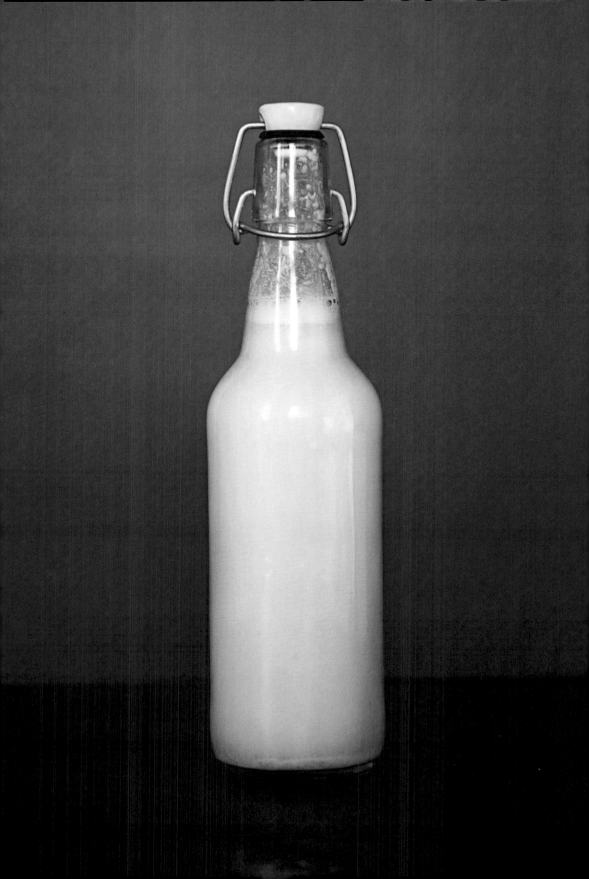

Cardamom nut milk

I like to drink this Middle Eastern-inspired milk
warm in the evening.

MAKES ABOUT 1 LITRE/1¾ PINTS/GENEROUS 4 CUPS

140g/5oz/1 cup shelled unsalted pistachio nuts, soaked,
drained and rinsed (see page 20)

1 litre/1¾ pints/generous 4 cups hot water

4 tbsp maple syrup

½ tsp sea salt

½ tsp cardamom seeds, crushed

Put all the ingredients in a blender and blend for 2–3 minutes
until smooth. Pour the contents into a nut bag, placed in a bowl.
Twist the bag to squeeze the liquid into the bowl and leave
to cool.

Pour the milk into a clean bottle with a tight-fitting lid. Place in
the fridge and leave to stand for a couple of hours or overnight
before using. Store in the fridge and use within 2 days.

Strawberry cashew milk

A nice base for smoothies or for pouring over some fresh berries in the summer.

MAKES ABOUT 1 LITRE/1¾ PINTS/GENEROUS 4 CUPS

185g/6½ oz/1½ cups cashew nuts, soaked, drained and rinsed (see page 20)

2 tsp maple syrup

½ tsp ground cinnamon

a pinch of sea salt

1 litre/1¾ pints/generous 4 cups water

100g/3½ oz/1 cup strawberries, hulled

Put all the ingredients, except the strawberries, in a blender and blend for 2–3 minutes until smooth. Add the strawberries towards the end and blend until the mixture is smooth. Pour the contents into a nut bag, placed in a bowl. Twist the bag to squeeze the liquid into the bowl.

Pour the milk into a clean bottle with a tight-fitting lid. Place in the fridge and leave to stand for a couple of hours or overnight before using. Store in the fridge and use within 2 days.

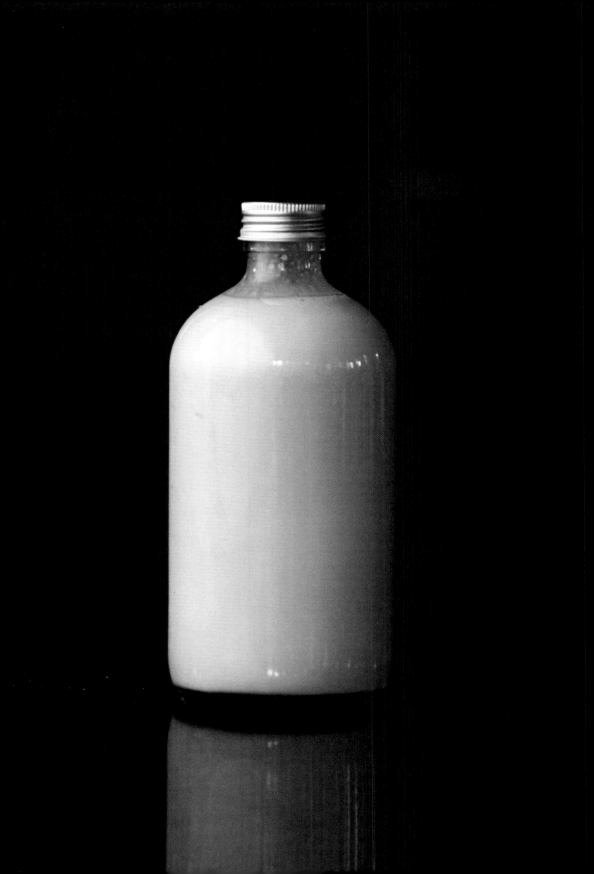

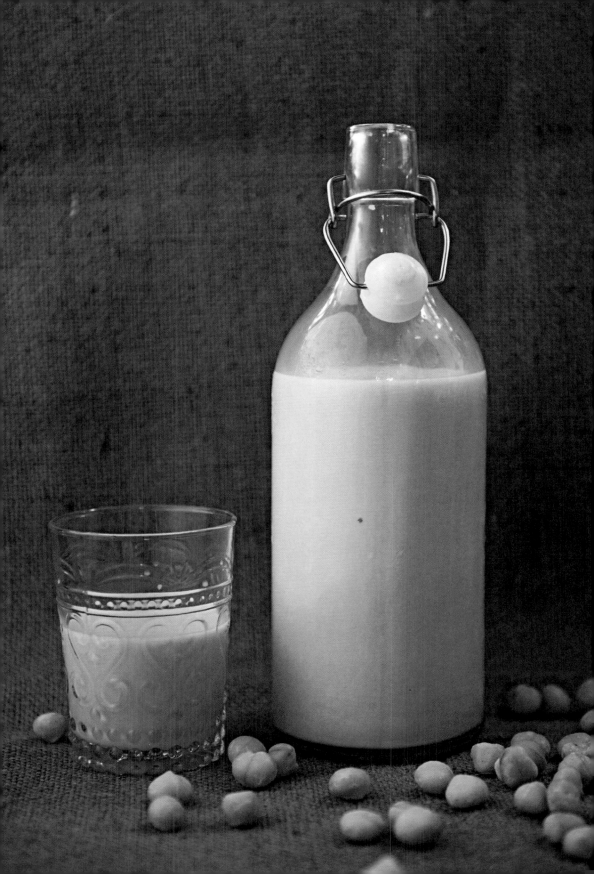

Macadamia milk

This milk has a creamy flavour, which makes it suitable as a base for ice cream. Make sure to blend the macadamias thoroughly, since they can be more difficult to grind than other nuts.

MAKES ABOUT 1 LITRE/1¾ PINTS/GENEROUS 4 CUPS

175g/6oz/scant 1½ cups macadamia nuts, soaked, drained and rinsed (see page 20)

1.2 litres/2 pints/5 cups hot water

a little sea salt

½ tsp vanilla powder

Put all the ingredients in a blender and blend on the highest speed for 2–3 minutes until smooth. Pour the contents into a nut bag, placed in a bowl. Twist the bag to squeeze the liquid into the bowl and leave to cool.

Pour the milk into a clean bottle with a tight-fitting lid. Store in the fridge and use within 3 days.

Pumpkin seed milk

A protein-rich super seed! When making milk from pumpkin seeds you also get a nice colour. Pumpkin seed milk is good for breakfast, in smoothies or in a pancake batter.

MAKES ABOUT 800ML/28FL OZ/3¼ CUPS

200g/7oz/scant 1½ cups pumpkin seeds, soaked, drained and rinsed (see page 20)

800ml/28fl oz/3¼ cups hot water

a pinch of sea salt

½ tsp vanilla powder

3 medjool dates, pitted and chopped

Put all the ingredients in a blender and blend for 1–2 minutes until smooth. Pour the contents into a nut bag, placed in a bowl. Twist the bag to squeeze the liquid into the bowl and leave to cool.

Pour the milk into a clean bottle with a tight-fitting lid. Place in the fridge and leave to stand for a couple of hours or overnight before using. Store in the fridge and use within 3–4 days.

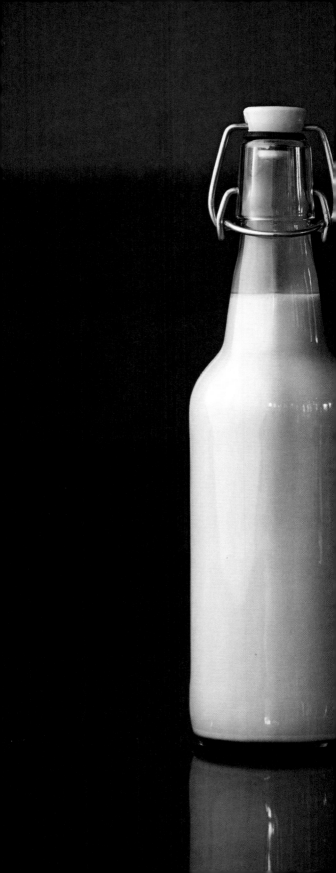

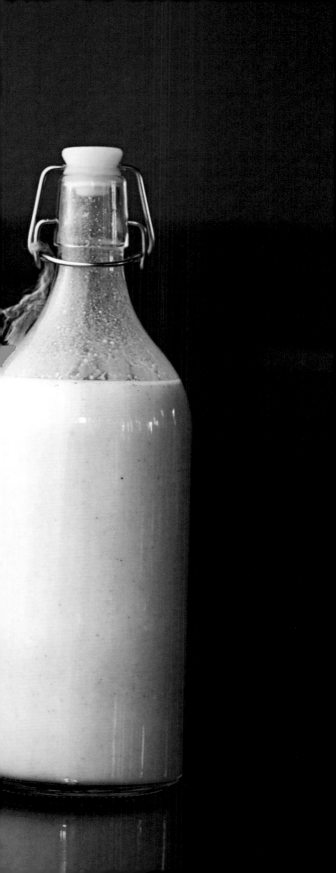

Hemp seed milk

Shelled hemp seeds are so soft that you don't need to separate the pulp from the liquid and they also give a pleasing whiteness to the milk. Hemp seed milk can be drunk plain, or it makes a good base for baking or cooking since it has a neutral flavour and is rich in nutrients. I like to drink it in the morning, preferably at room temperature, to slowly awaken the stomach.

MAKES ABOUT 1 LITRE/1¾ PINTS/GENEROUS 4 CUPS

½ vanilla pod

1 litre/1¾ pints/generous 4 cups water

175g/6oz/1¼ cups shelled hemp seeds

a pinch of sea salt

Cut the vanilla pod lengthways and scrape out the seeds. Put the vanilla seeds, water, hemp seeds and salt in a blender and blend for 1 minute.

Pour the milk into a clean bottle with a tight-fitting lid. Store in the fridge and use within 4 days.

Pistachio and spirulina milk

What I like about pistachio nuts is not just their lovely colour but also their flavour. In this recipe, I've added a little spirulina powder to give the milk an extra green colour. Add the spirulina once the milk has cooled to retain its nutrients. Use the milk in ice cream or smoothies.

MAKES ABOUT 1 LITRE/1¾ PINTS/GENEROUS 4 CUPS

185g/6½ oz/1⅓ cups shelled unsalted pistachio nuts, soaked, drained and rinsed (see page 20)
1 litre/1¾ pints/generous 4 cups hot water
4 medjool dates, pitted and chopped
1 tbsp spirulina powder

Put the nuts, water and dates in a blender and blend on the highest speed for 2–3 minutes until smooth. Pour the contents into a nut bag, placed in a bowl. Twist the bag to squeeze the liquid into the bowl and leave to cool.

Pour the milk back into the blender, add the spirulina powder and blend for a further 1 minute.

Pour the milk into a clean bottle with a tight-fitting lid. Store in the fridge and use within 2–3 days.

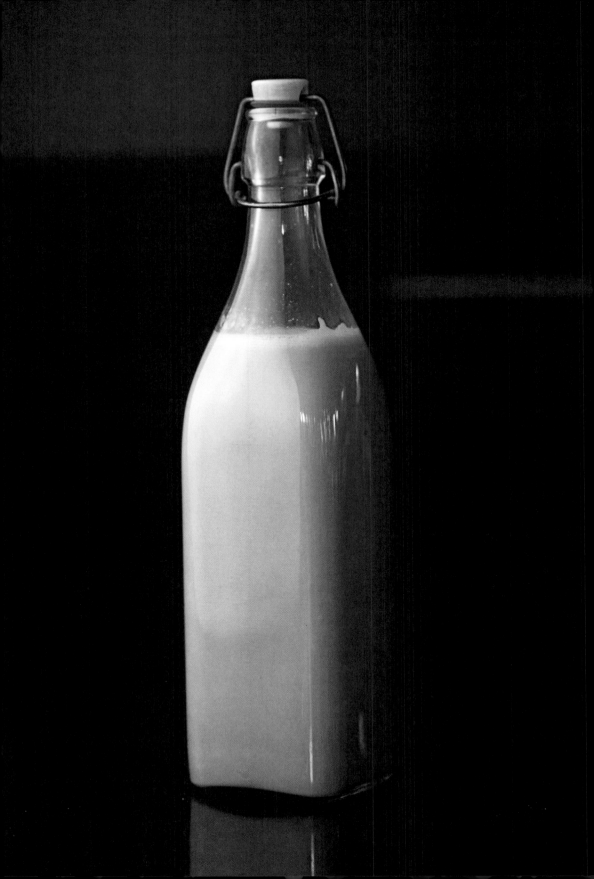

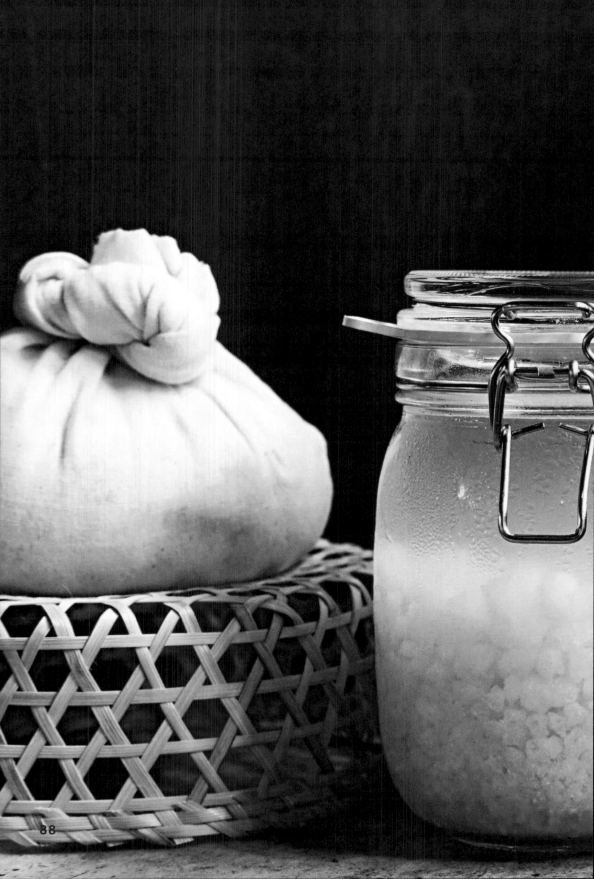

Yogurt, cream & cheese

Now the fun begins! These vegan versions of yogurt, cream and cheese are made through the fermentation of nuts. You'll need a little patience and time – planning is also key – but it's so rewarding to be able to serve homemade vegan cheese or cream and eat your own yogurt in the morning, that it's really worth the effort.

Coconut yogurt

If you're making yogurt for the first time I recommend this recipe since it's so easy. It uses canned coconut milk, which you can get in any supermarket. The yogurt is perfect for breakfast or it can be added to a smoothie.

MAKES ABOUT 200ML/ 7FL OZ/SCANT 1 CUP

400ml/14fl oz can organic coconut milk, at room temperature

²/₃ tsp powder or 2 capsules good-quality probiotics

vanilla powder or maple syrup, to taste

Pour the coconut milk into a bowl and whisk until smooth. Add the probiotic powder and whisk until mixed in.

Pour into a clean glass jar and cover with clingfilm (plastic wrap) or a cloth. Leave to stand at room temperature out of direct sunlight for about 24 hours.

Taste the yogurt – it should be a little sour when ready with small air bubbles on the surface. Leave to stand for up to a further 12 hours if it's not.

When the yogurt is ready, add a little vanilla or maple syrup to taste.

Seal the jar with a tight-fitting lid. Store in the fridge and use within 1 week.

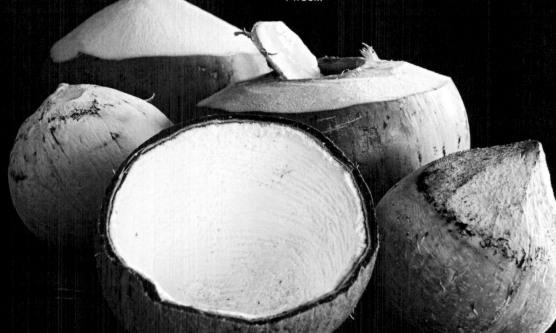

Coconut kefir

Coconut kefir is a yogurt-like drink and is delicious served on its own or added to smoothies.

MAKES ABOUT 400ML/ 14FL OZ/1¾ CUPS

300ml/10fl oz/1¼ cups
   hot water
150g/5½ oz/2 cups
   desiccated (shredded)
   coconut
3 tbsp maple syrup
3 tbsp Water Kefir (see
   page 13)
½ tsp vanilla powder or
   extra maple syrup

Add the water and coconut to a blender and blend for 3–5 minutes until smooth.

Line a bowl with muslin (cheesecloth) and pour in the coconut mixture. Gather up the sides of the cloth and squeeze the liquid into the bowl, then discard the pulp. Stir in the syrup with a wooden or plastic spoon and leave to stand until the milk cools to room temperature.

Add the water kefir and stir until mixed in. Pour into a clean glass jar and cover with clingfilm (plastic wrap) or a cloth. Leave to stand at room temperature out of direct sunlight for 12–24 hours.

Taste the kefir – it should be a little sour when ready with small air bubbles on the surface. Leave to stand for up to a further 12 hours if it's not, checking and tasting the kefir occasionally.

When the kefir is ready, add the vanilla powder or extra syrup to taste.

Seal the jar with a tight-fitting lid. Store in the fridge and use within 1 week.

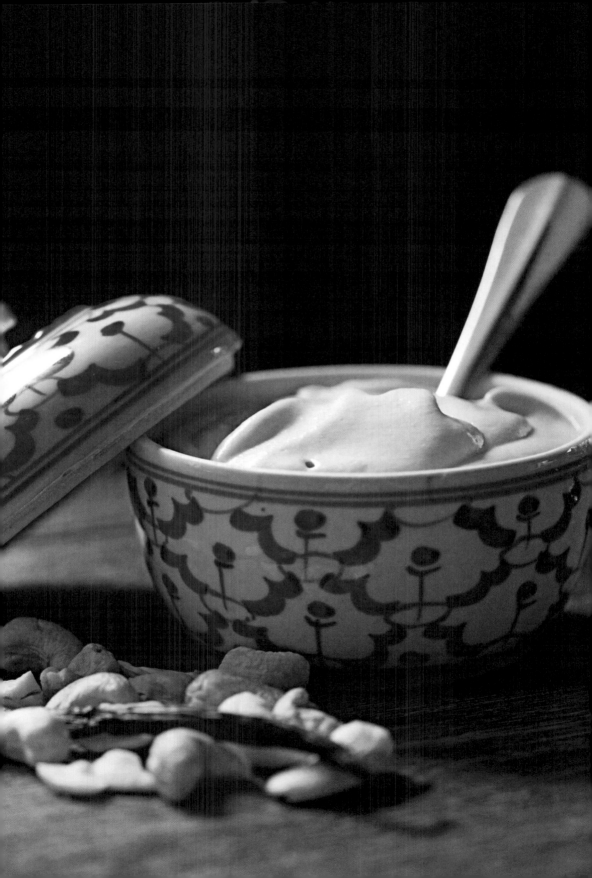

Cashew cream

The cashew is a fantastic nut and makes a delicious vegan alternative to cream. This version is a great all-rounder, use it in desserts or any dish where you need whipped cream.

SERVES ABOUT 4

280g/10oz/2¼ cups cashew nuts, soaked, drained and rinsed (see page 20)

a pinch of sea salt

¼ tsp vanilla powder

5 tbsp maple syrup

1 tbsp lemon juice

200–300ml/7–10fl oz/scant 1 cup–1¼ cups water, to taste

Put all the ingredients, except the water, in a blender. Pulse while gradually adding the water, using the smaller quantity for a thicker cream and adding more if you like.

Leave the blender to run on the highest speed for 2–3 minutes until the mixture has a fluffy cream-like consistency.

Serve immediately.

Quick cashew yogurt

A quick, tasty and nutritious breakfast yogurt. Enjoy with granola and berries.

SERVES ABOUT 4

1 recipe quantity of Cashew Cream (see page 93)
juice of ½ lemon
juice of ½ orange
½ tsp vanilla powder

Whisk together all the ingredients in a bowl. If the consistency is too thick, dilute it with a little water.

Serve immediately.

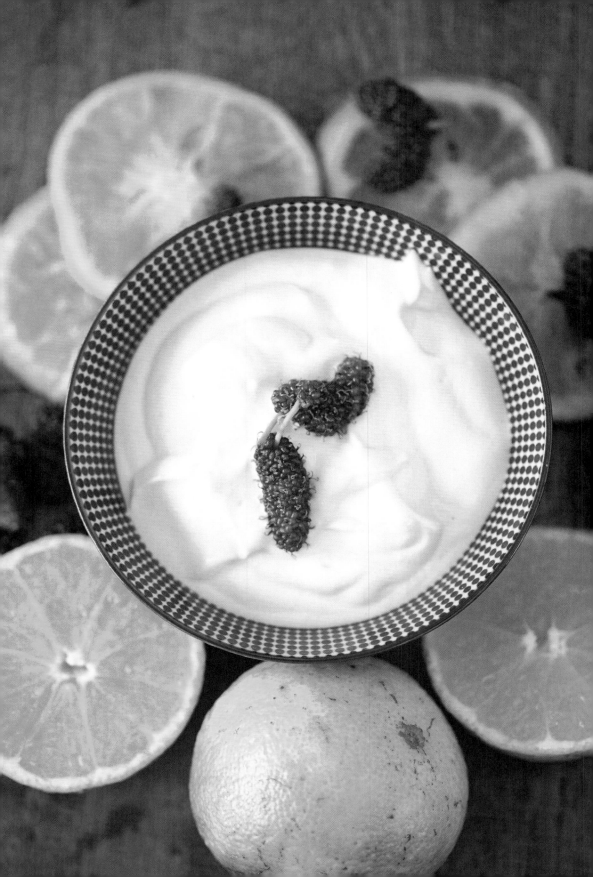

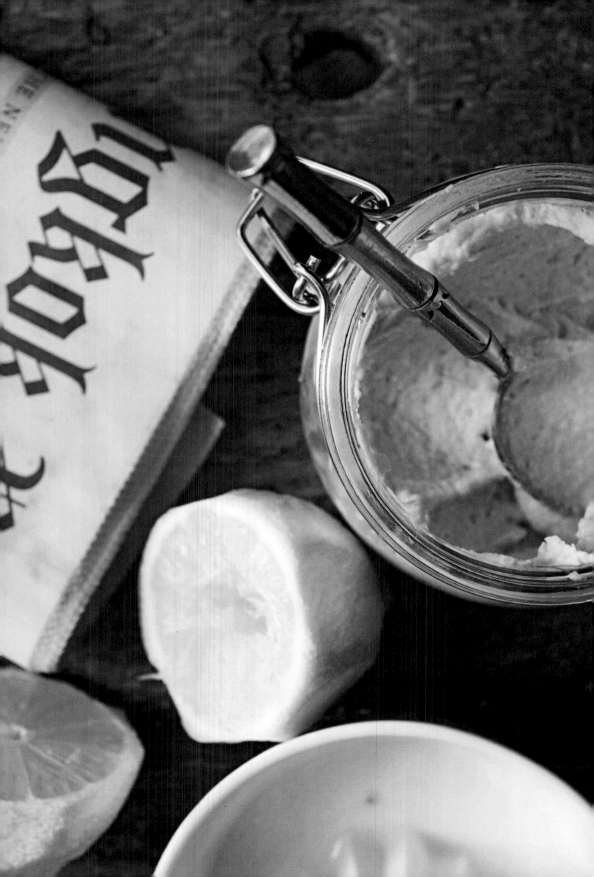

Cashew yogurt with live cultures

This amazing yogurt does the body a whole lot of good! The added probiotics or live cultures help to boost the health of the gut and the immune system.

SERVES ABOUT 6

475g/1lb 1oz/4 cups cashew nuts, soaked, drained and rinsed (see page 20)

400ml/14fl oz/scant 1¾ cups water

4 tbsp lemon juice

a pinch of sea salt

1 tsp powder or 3 capsules good-quality probiotics

Put all the ingredients, except the probiotics, in a blender and blend to a smooth, thick cream. Transfer to a bowl, add the probiotic powder and mix thoroughly.

Cover the bowl with a cloth, move it to a cool place out of direct sunlight and leave to stand overnight or for 12 hours until thickened and it tastes a little sour.

Pour the yogurt into a clean jar with a tight-fitting lid. Store in the fridge and use within 4 days.

TIP

You can sweeten the yogurt with a spoonful of Date Caramel Paste (see page 140).

Vanilla coconut cream

Sometimes the simplest ideas are the best! If you have a can of coconut milk to hand, then this couldn't be easier to make. Use the cream in desserts and cakes or spooned over fruit and berries.

SERVES ABOUT 4

400ml/14fl oz can organic coconut milk

⅓ tsp vanilla powder

Chill the unopened can of coconut milk in the fridge for at least 1 hour. Open the can from the bottom and pour away the watery liquid (save it for another recipe).

Spoon the solidified coconut cream into a mixing bowl. Add the vanilla and beat with an electric whisk for a few minutes until thick and creamy.

Serve immediately or store in a sealed jar in the fridge and use within 2–3 days.

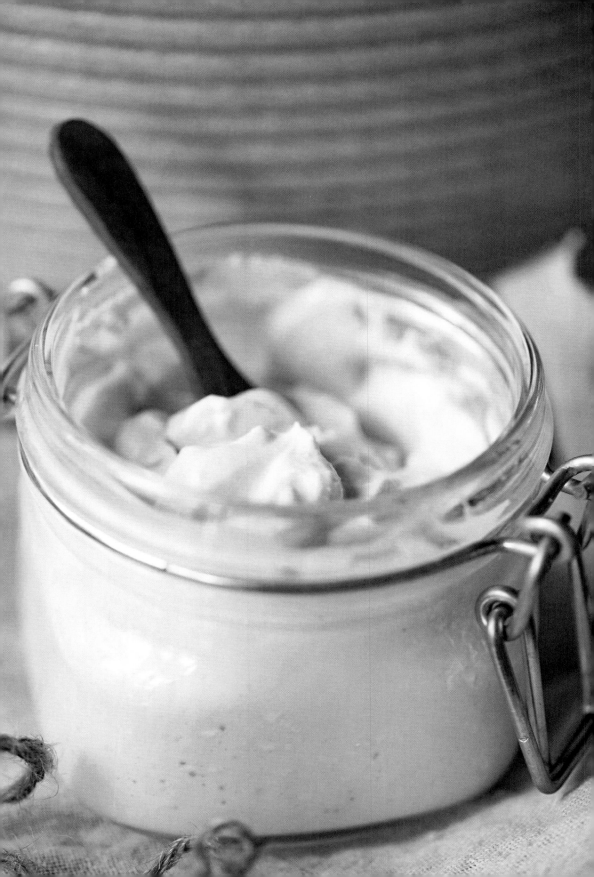

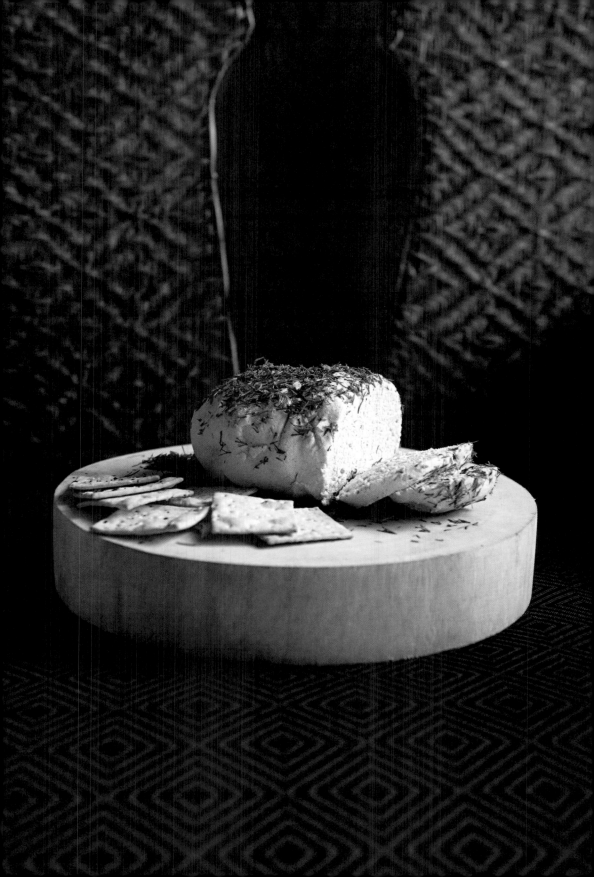

Fresh dill cheese

Choosing which flavourings to add to your homemade vegan cheese is a question of taste. Here, I've used fresh dill as a topping. This cheese makes a great addition to a cheeseboard, served with crackers and nibbles.

SERVES 4-6

185g/6½ oz/1½ cups cashew nuts, soaked, drained and rinsed (see page 20)
2 tbsp nutritional yeast flakes
2 tbsp lemon juice
1 tsp cider vinegar
1 tsp garlic powder or 1 garlic clove, crushed
½ tsp sea salt
½ tsp freshly ground black pepper
2 tbsp water
⅔ tsp or 2 capsules good-quality probiotics
chopped fresh dill, to garnish

Put the nuts, nutritional yeast flakes, lemon juice, vinegar, garlic, salt, pepper and water in a blender and blend for 5 minutes or until smooth and creamy. If the mixture is difficult to work, add an extra spoonful or two of water.

Transfer the mixture to a bowl, add the probiotic powder and stir with a plastic or wooden spoon. Cover and leave to stand in the fridge for a couple of hours. Alternatively, spoon the mixture into a cheese bag. Twist the bag to shape the mixture into a ball and place it in a colander over a bowl. Cover and leave to stand in the fridge overnight.

To serve, remove the bowl from the fridge or unwrap the cheese and place it on a plate. Season to taste with extra salt and pepper and sprinkle the dill over the top.

Cover and store in the fridge and eat within 3 days.

Almond cheese

When making nut cheese, almond is a good one to start with. This base recipe works well as a spreadable cheese on bread, but if you'd like a harder cheese, leave it at room temperature until firmed up (see page 105).

SERVES 4-6

375g/13oz/2¾ cups almonds, soaked, drained and rinsed (see page 20)

3–6 tbsp Water Kefir (see page 13), just enough to blend the nuts

a pinch of sea salt

Add the almonds to a blender with the smaller quantity of kefir and the salt and blend to a smooth cream. If the mixture is difficult to work, add some more of the kefir.

Spoon the cream into a clean bowl, cover with a cloth and secure with an elastic band. Leave to stand at room temperature for 24–48 hours. It's ready when the cheese thickens slightly and tastes a little sour.

Store in the fridge and eat within 10 days.

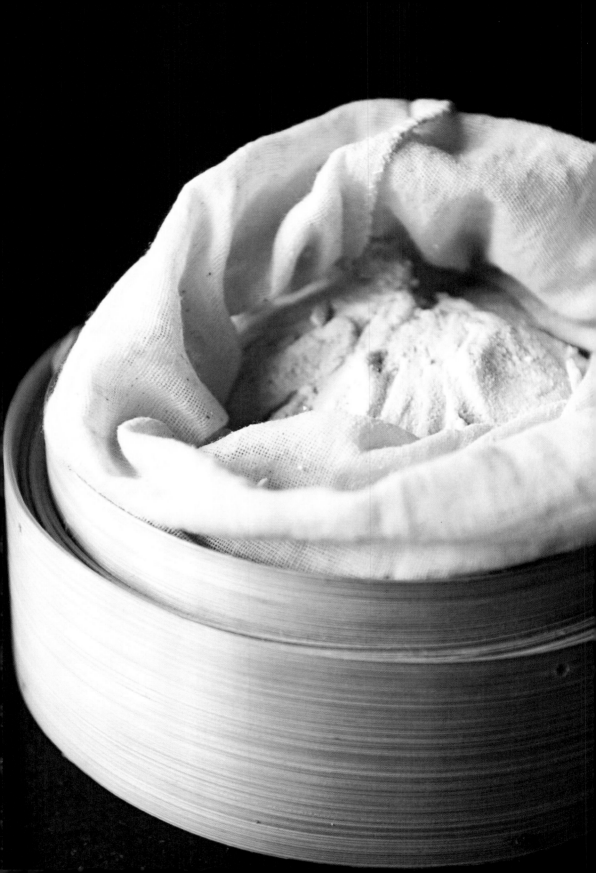

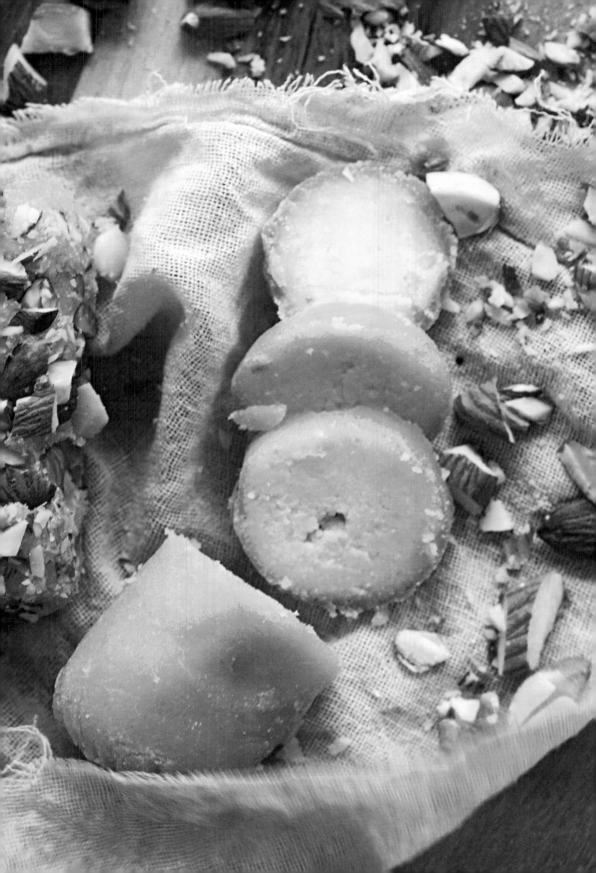

Hard almond cheese

This hard cheese develops a rind during maturing and is similar to a dairy cheese in flavour. I like to eat it with sesame seed crackers.

SERVES 4-6

1 recipe quantity of Almond
   Cheese (see page 102)
1 tbsp nutritional yeast flakes
1 tbsp white miso paste
1 tsp sea salt, plus extra for
   maturing

Blend all the ingredients together until smooth. Place a piece of muslin (cheesecloth) in a small bowl and add the almond mixture.

Gather the cloth around the almond mixture to form it into a ball and secure the top with an elastic band or string. Salt the ball from the outside of the cloth to protect the cheese from going mouldy. Place the ball in a colander over a bowl and leave to stand at room temperature for 2 days.

When ready, carefully remove the cloth from the cheese. Shape the cheese and salt the surface. It can be eaten straight away, but if you'd like a smoother flavour and more rind, cover with a cloth and leave it to stand at room temperature for an additional couple of days.

Wrap the cheese in waxed paper or clingfilm (plastic wrap). Store in the fridge and eat within 10 days.

Parmesan seed cheese

A super simple and quick recipe for parmesan seed cheese to use in salads, dressings, on pasta or any other dish where you'd like a nutty cheesy flavour.

SERVES ABOUT 4

150g/5½ oz/scant 1¼ cups sunflower seeds
4 tbsp nutritional yeast flakes
½ tsp onion powder
1 tsp smoked paprika
1 tsp sea salt

Toast the sunflower seeds in a dry frying pan (skillet) until light golden. Leave to cool.

Add all the ingredients to a blender or food processor and pulse until coarsely chopped.

Store in the fridge in an airtight container. It will keep for several weeks.

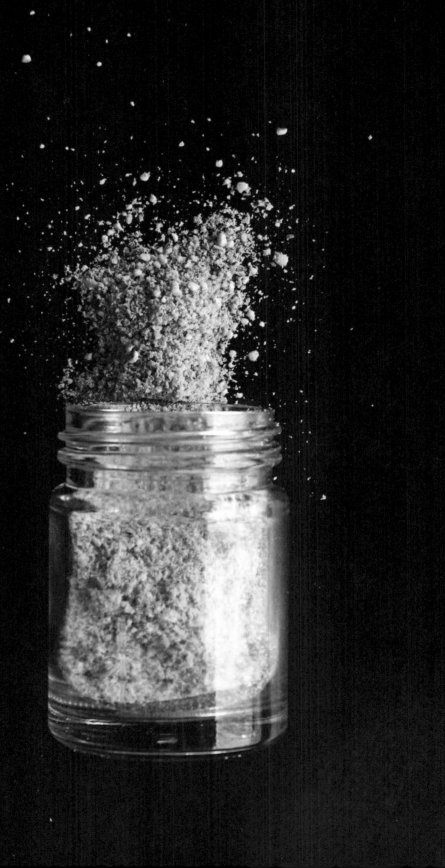

Ricotta nut cheese

I really like this vegan version of ricotta cheese. It's a good alternative to butter made from cow's milk since it's so easy to spread onto bread. Enjoy with a sprinkle of fresh herbs, shoots, seeds and vegetables.

SERVES 4-6

350g/12oz/scant 3 cups macadamia nuts, soaked, drained and rinsed (see page 20)

100ml/3½ fl oz/generous ⅓ cup water

juice of ½ lemon

a pinch of sea salt

Put all the ingredients in a food processor and blend until smooth and creamy. Spoon the cheese into a bowl.

Cover and store in the fridge and eat within 5 days.

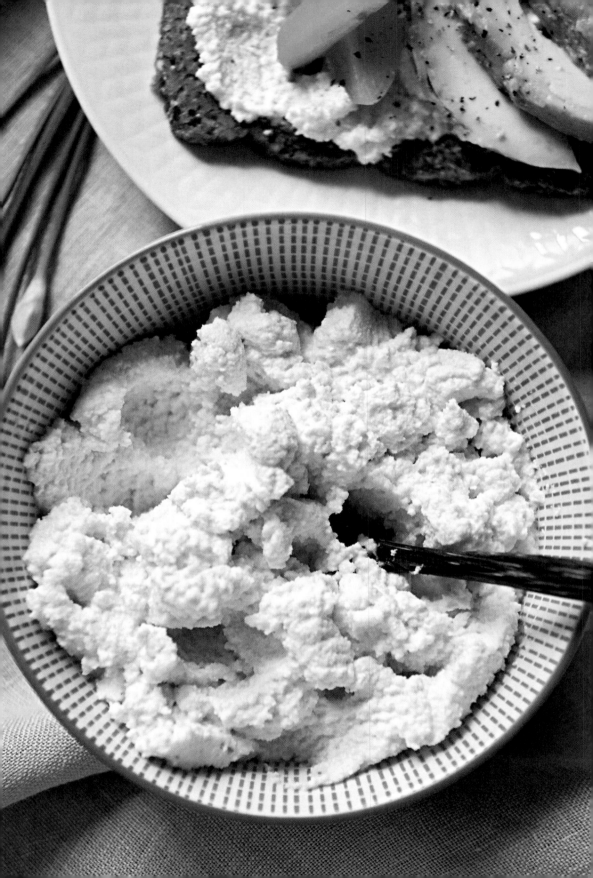

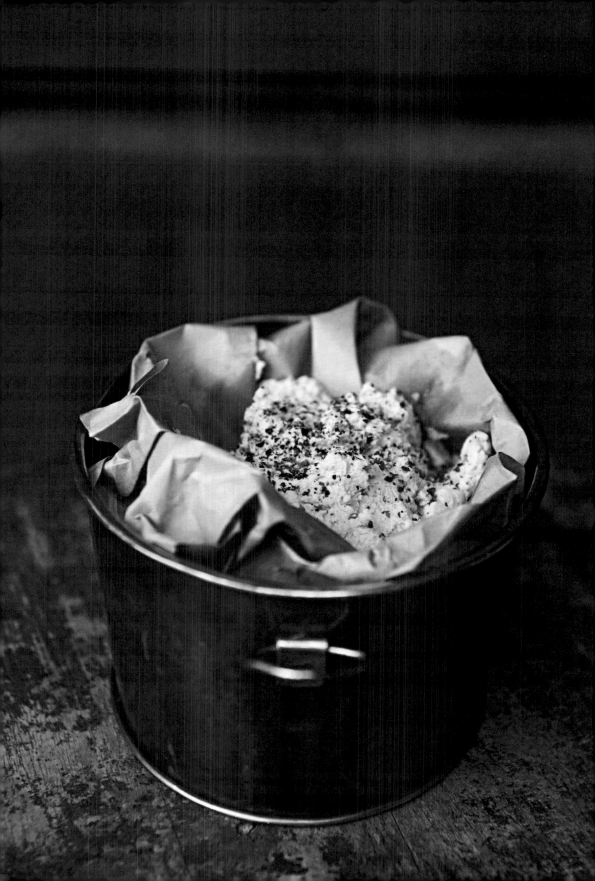

Soft cheese
with roasted garlic

A spicy and flavourful cheese that tastes wonderful. I like to add
a few chunks to my salad or enjoy on a cracker.

SERVES 4-6

2 garlic cloves
185g/6½ oz/1½ cups cashew
 nuts, soaked, drained and
 rinsed (see page 20)
2 tbsp nutritional yeast flakes
2 tbsp lemon juice
1 tsp cider vinegar
½ tsp sea salt
½ tsp freshly ground black
 pepper
2 tbsp water
⅔ tsp powder or 2 capsules
 good-quality probiotics
crushed red or pink peppercorns and black pepper,
 to garnish

Preheat the oven to 200°C/400°F/
Gas Mark 6. Put the garlic in a roasting
tin (pan) and roast for 15–20 minutes
until golden. Remove from the oven and
leave to cool.

Put the cashews, nutritional yeast flakes,
lemon juice, vinegar, garlic, salt, pepper
and water in a blender and blend for
5 minutes until smooth and creamy. If the
mixture is difficult to work, add an extra
spoonful or two of water.

Transfer the mixture to a bowl, add the
probiotic powder and stir with a plastic
or wooden spoon. Cover and leave to
stand in the fridge for a couple of hours.
Alternatively, spoon the mixture into
a cheese bag. Twist the bag to shape
the mixture into a ball and place it in a
colander over a bowl. Cover and leave
to stand in the fridge overnight.

To serve, remove the bowl from the
fridge or unwrap the cheese and place
it on a plate. Sprinkle over extra salt, the
crushed peppercorns and black pepper.

Cover and store in the fridge and eat
within 3 days.

Hard cashew cheese

Hard cashew cheese has to be matured for 10–14 days in the fridge before it is ready to eat. Shape it into a long rectangle or roll so that you can easily cut it into slices. If you want to flavour the cheese, do so while it's fermenting. My flavour suggestions include chilli, garlic, paprika or powdered onion – simply add about ½ teaspoon of your choice of flavouring and taste. To make the cheese look prettier, you can roll it in fresh herbs after it has matured.

SERVES 4-6

350g/12oz/scant 3 cups cashew
   nuts, soaked, drained
   and rinsed (see page 20)
about 6–7 tbsp water
2–3 tsp powder or 6–9 capsules
   good-quality probiotics
1 tsp sea salt
2 tbsp nutritional yeast flakes
1 tbsp lemon juice

Blend the cashews for 5 minutes in a blender with 3 tablespoons water, adding more when needed until a thick, creamy consistency – you don't want it to be too wet. Occasionally stir the mixture if your blender is struggling.

Transfer the cream to a bowl and stir in the probiotic powder using a plastic or wooden spoon. Cover with a cloth or baking (parchment) paper and leave to stand at room temperature for 1–2 days, depending on how fermented you like it.

When the cheese has an acidic flavour and you think it has fermented enough, add the salt, nutritional yeast flakes and lemon juice and mix thoroughly using a plastic or wooden spoon.

Spoon the cheese into a long sausage or rectangular shape on a sheet of baking paper, about 30 x 10cm/12 x 4 inches. Roll the paper tightly around the cheese, pressing it to make a long roulade or rectangle and fold the ends under. Leave the cheese to firm up and mature in the fridge for 10–14 days – although it can be eaten before this.

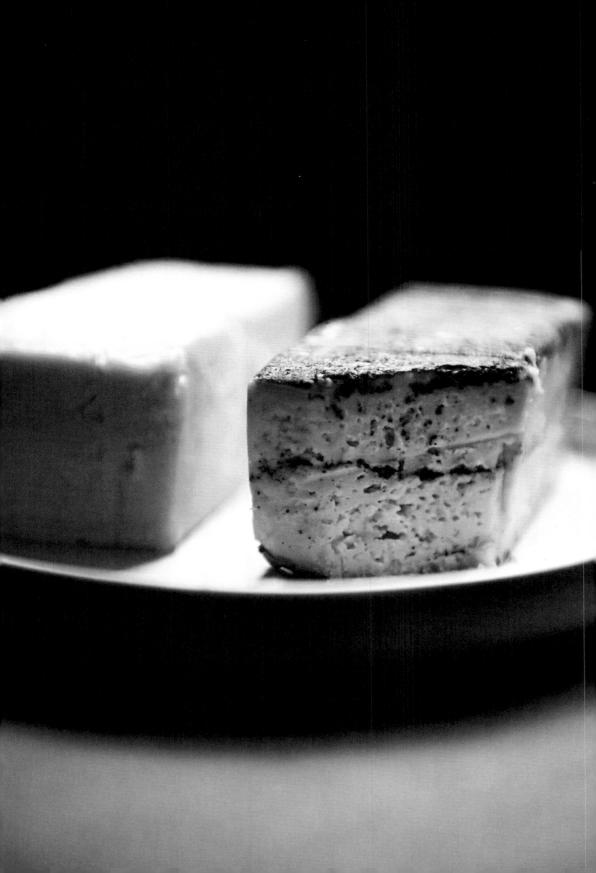

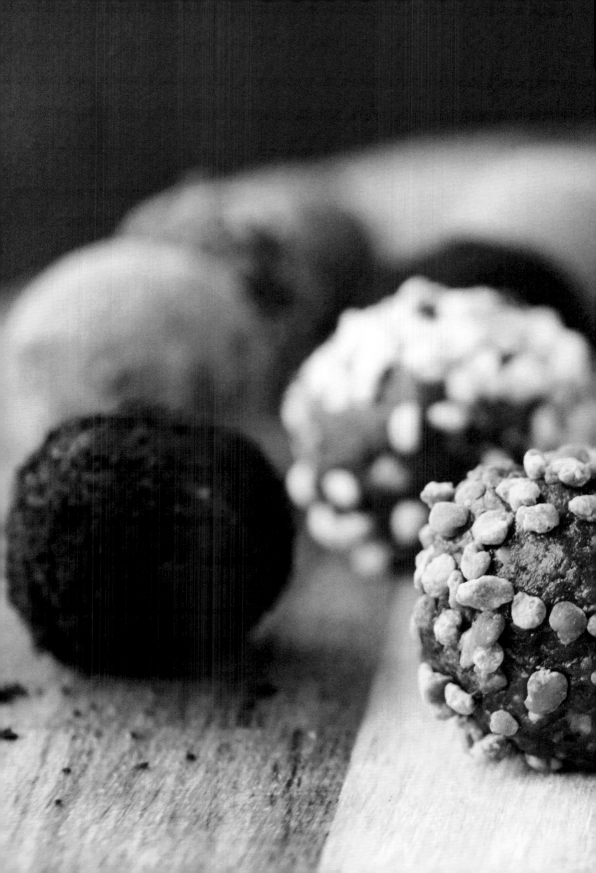

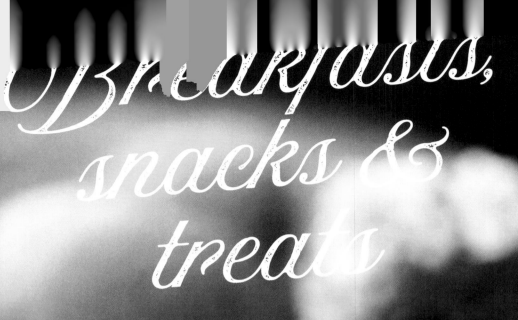

Breakfasts, snacks & treats

All of the recipes up until now can be used as an ingredient
in other recipes. And to show you just how versatile they are,
I've gathered a selection of sweet and savoury vegan dishes
that use some of the recipes given earlier in the book.
Since we've saved so much pulp from the nut milk
chapter, I've included a recipe for using it up as well.
You'll also find recipes for snacks and treats that
are delicious eaten with vegan dairy products.

Sesame seed crispbread

Of course you'd want some nice crispbread to serve with your home-made vegan cheese, aubergine (eggplant) dip or hummus, right? This recipe is quick and easy to make and contains just six ingredients.

SERVES ABOUT 4

140g/5oz/heaped 1 cup gram (chickpea) flour
1 tbsp black sesame seeds
1 tsp bicarbonate of soda (baking soda)
½ tsp sea salt
1 tsp coconut oil, melted
2 tbsp water

Preheat the oven to 200°C/400°F/Gas Mark 6.

Mix together the dry ingredients in a bowl and add the oil and water. Mix with your hands until it forms a dough.

Place the dough on a large sheet of baking (parchment) paper. Put another sheet on top and roll out as thinly as possible. Remove the top sheet of paper and cut the dough using a knife or pizza cutter into squares, each about 7–8cm/2¾–3¼ inches.

Carefully lift the paper and dough squares onto a baking tray (sheet) and bake in the middle of the oven for 20 minutes or until crisp and golden.

Leave to cool on a wire rack. Serve immediately or store in an airtight tin and eat within 1–2 days.

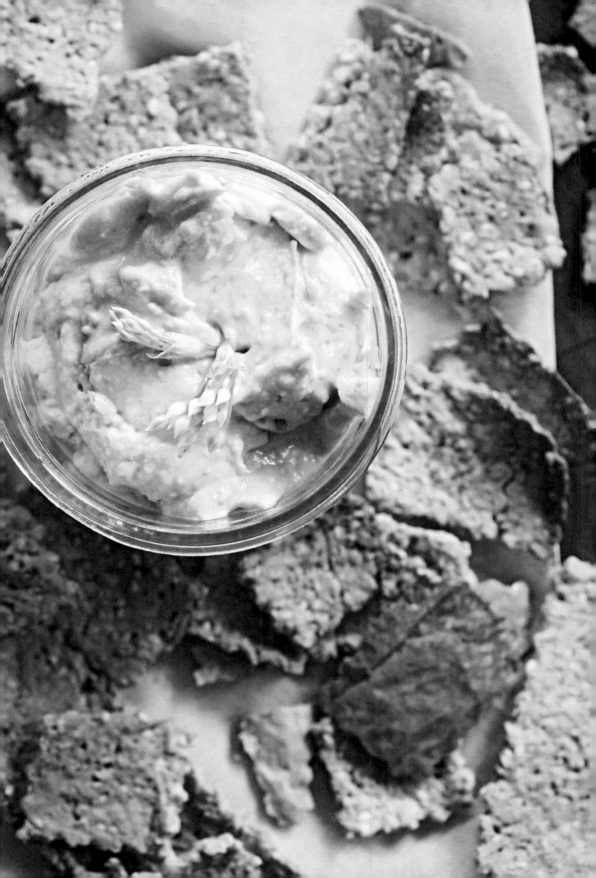

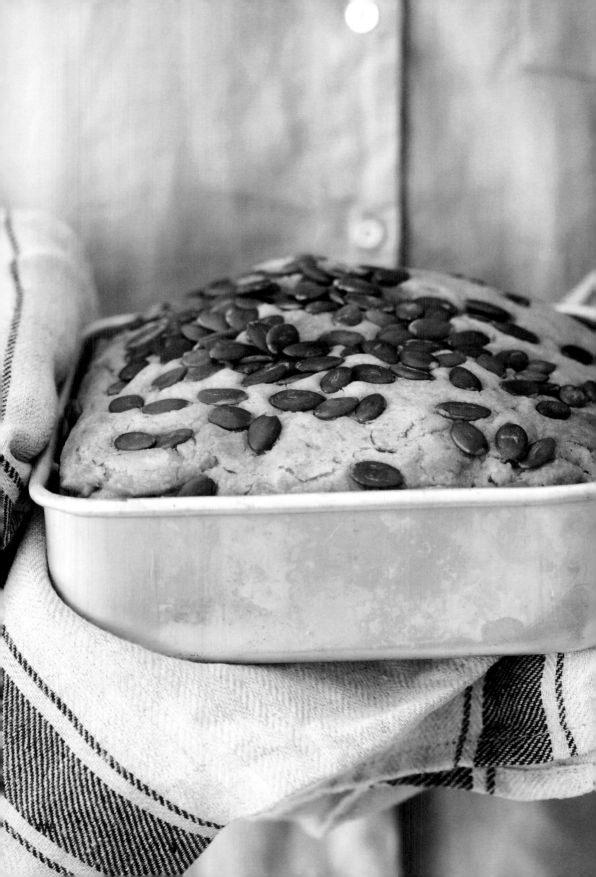

Chickpea bread

A simple recipe with few ingredients and a great way to use up hummus. This makes a flavourful and nutritious loaf that can be enjoyed at any time of the day. I recommend using buckwheat flour, but you can also try using gram (chickpea) flour or quinoa flour.

MAKES 1 LOAF

500g/1lb 2oz/generous 4 cups buckwheat flour

1½ tbsp bicarbonate of soda (baking soda)

400ml/14fl oz/scant 1¾ cups water

225g/8oz/1 cup Pepper Hummus (see page 123)

150g/5½ oz/scant ¾ cup Tahini (see page 40), or use ready-made

1 tsp sea salt

GARNISH:

pumpkin seeds

sea salt

Preheat the oven to 200°C/400°F/Gas Mark 6.

Mix all the ingredients together in a bowl. Grease a 900g/2lb loaf tin (pan) with oil or line with baking (parchment) paper. Pour the mixture into the loaf tin and top with pumpkin seeds and a sprinkling of salt.

Cover the tin with foil and bake for 1 hour or until risen and cooked through. Take the bread out of the oven and leave it to cool for a few minutes on a wire rack. Turn it out of the tin and leave to cool completely.

Cover and store and eat within 2–3 days.

Beetroot crisps
with rosemary

A perfect colourful snack to serve with baba ganoush, hummus or vegan nut cheese.

SERVES ABOUT 4

2 large or 3 medium-sized raw beetroots (beets)

sea salt

2–3 fresh rosemary sprigs

Slice the beetroots thinly into rounds using a mandolin or sharp knife. Arrange the slices on baking (parchment) paper, spreading them out evenly, and sprinkle with salt. Leave to stand for 30 minutes.

Preheat the oven to 180°C/350°F/Gas Mark 4.

Pat the beetroot slices dry and arrange them on baking paper-lined baking trays (sheets). Add the rosemary, tucking it in between the beetroot.

Bake for 20 minutes, turning the slices over halfway through, until crisp. Leave to cool and serve sprinkled with extra salt if needed. Serve and enjoy straight away.

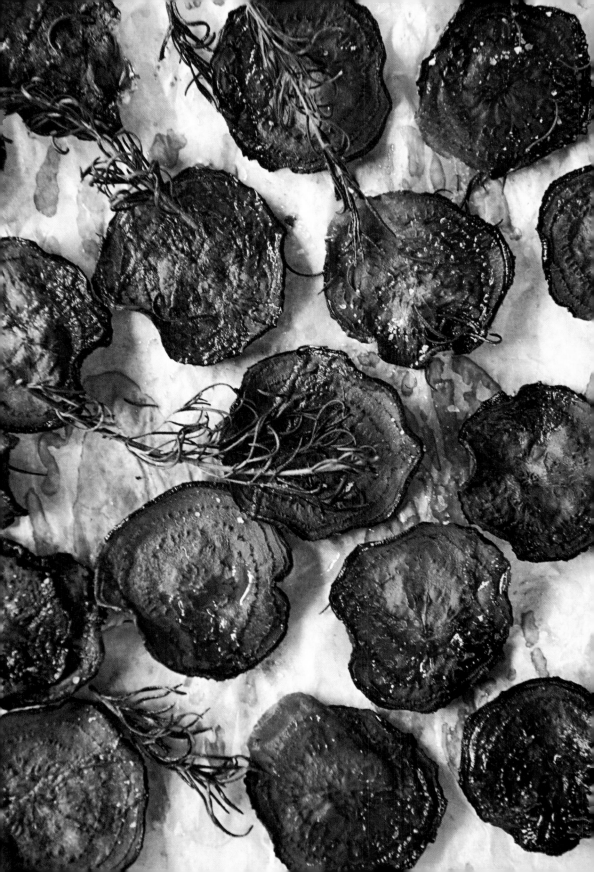

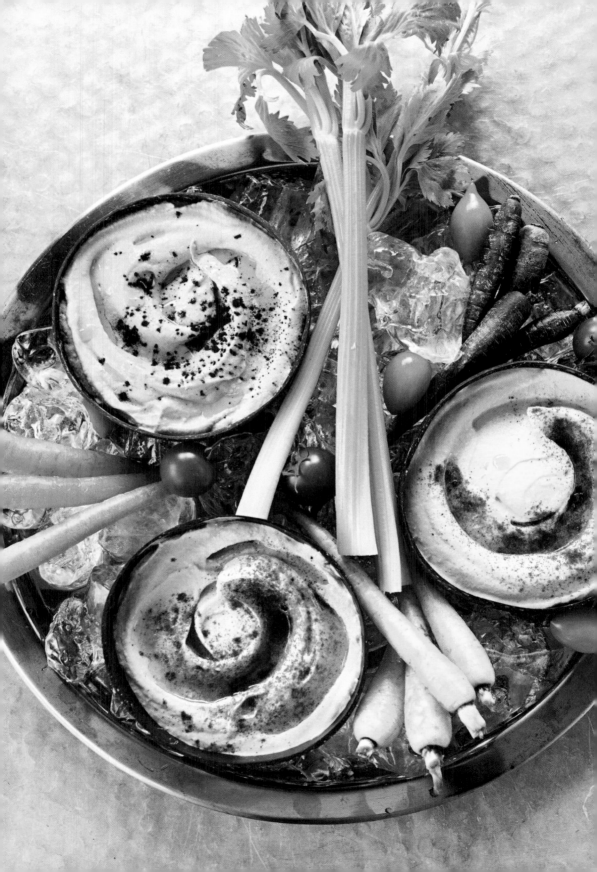

Pepper hummus

Hummus is so much more fun when it's brightly coloured! Make a batch of hummus and then add the (bell) pepper of your choice – red, yellow or green. Serve with cherry tomatoes and vegetable sticks.

SERVES ABOUT 4

400g/14oz can chickpeas,
  drained and rinsed
2 garlic cloves
1 red, yellow or green (bell)
  pepper, deseeded
1 tbsp lemon juice
3 tbsp Tahini (see page 40),
  or use ready-made
2 tbsp olive oil
½ tsp ground cumin
3 tbsp water

GARNISH:

olive oil
pine kernels
fresh herbs
paprika

Put all the ingredients, except the water, in a food processor. Blend, adding a little water at a time, until you're happy with the consistency and the hummus is smooth and creamy.

Spoon it into a bowl, drizzle over some olive oil and finish with a sprinkling of pine kernels, herbs and/or paprika.

Cover and store in the fridge and eat within 3–4 days.

Baba ganoush

To be completely honest, I don't particularly like aubergine (eggplant) that much, but I can never get enough of this dip! Tahini livens up all sorts of dishes and in combination with the spices, ensures this baba ganoush is a success. Serve it with crackers.

SERVES ABOUT 4

1 large aubergine (eggplant)
olive oil, for brushing
4 tbsp Tahini (see page 40), or use ready-made
1 tbsp olive oil
3 garlic cloves, finely chopped
a pinch of ground cumin
a pinch of cayenne pepper
juice of 1 lemon
a pinch of sea salt

GARNISH:

olive oil
fresh thyme sprigs
sesame seeds

Brush the aubergine with oil and then prick holes all over it using a skewer.

Cook the aubergine in a griddle pan over a high heat, turning it occasionally to make sure it cooks evenly. After 15 minutes, test if the aubergine is cooked by piercing it with a knife – it's ready when the knife goes in easily and the skin is charred. If it's not ready, continue to cook it, then test again. Leave to cool.

Remove the skin and cut the aubergine into chunks. Add the aubergine to a food processor and pulse a couple of times. Add the tahini and oil. Pulse again until all the ingredients are mixed together, then blend until smooth and creamy. Add the garlic, cumin, cayenne pepper and lemon juice and blend. Add salt to taste.

To serve, spoon the baba ganoush into a bowl, drizzle over a little oil and sprinkle with thyme and sesame seeds.

Cover and store in the fridge and eat within 3–4 days.

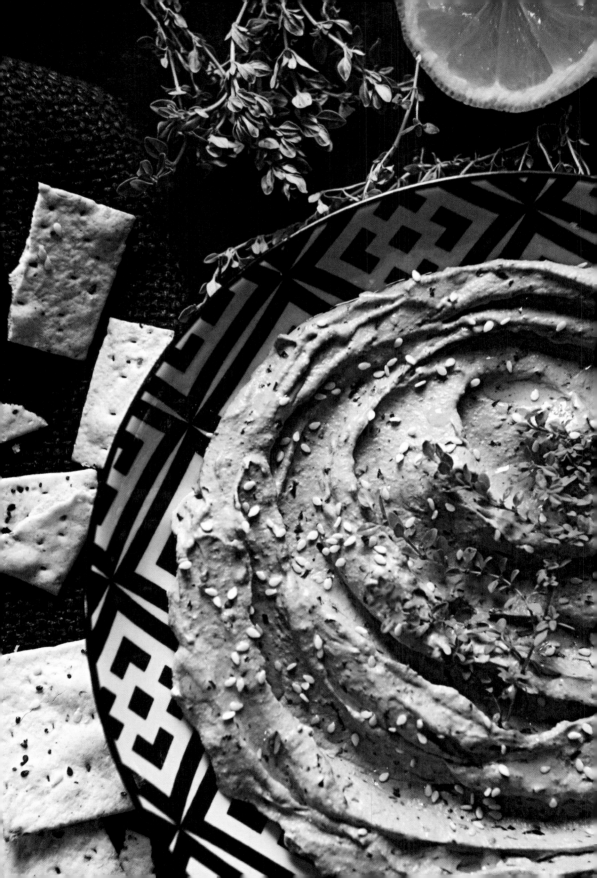

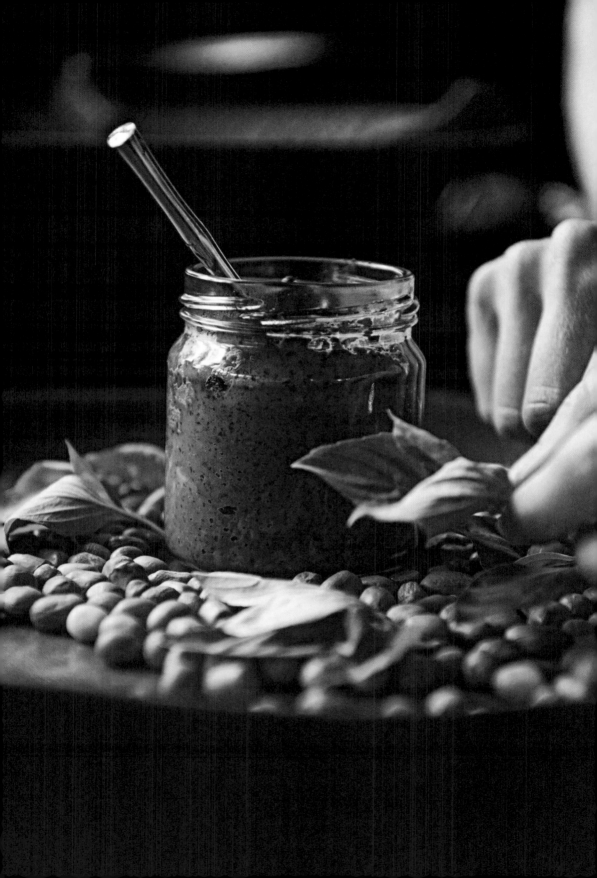

Thai pesto

This fragrant pesto works as a dip or dressing, or it can be stirred into creamy coconut sauces, vegan soft cheese, cooked pasta or egg noodles. For a hot Thai pesto, add some chopped fresh green chilli.

SERVES ABOUT 4

1 large bunch of Thai basil, leaves only

70g/2½ oz/¾ cup unsalted peanuts, toasted

4 tbsp sesame oil

2 garlic cloves

1 tbsp coconut sugar

1 tbsp rice vinegar or cider vinegar

1 tsp soy sauce or tamari

Put all the ingredients in a blender or food processor and blend on the highest speed until smooth.

Spoon the pesto into a clean glass jar with a tight-fitting lid. Store in the fridge and use within 4–5 days.

Peanut and banana ice cream

'Kind ice cream' is what we call ice cream that is made using bananas. This version is actually very kind to the stomach since it contains yogurt with active bacterial cultures. If you want to skip the yogurt, you can use your favourite nut milk instead.

SERVES 2-4

4 ripe bananas, peeled, cut
  into chunks and frozen
250g/9oz/generous 1 cup
  Peanut Butter (see page 36),
  plus extra to serve
3 tbsp nut yogurt of your
  choice, or nut milk
2 tsp maca powder
100g/3½ oz plain chocolate,
  finely chopped or use chips

TOPPING:

2-4 tbsp chopped nuts
  of your choice,
toasted 2-4 tbsp coconut
  flakes (chips)

Put the frozen bananas, peanut butter, yogurt or milk and maca into a blender and blend on the highest speed for a few minutes until the bananas have thawed and the mixture is creamy.

Add the dark chocolate towards the end and blend on a low speed for 1 minute until the ice cream is thoroughly mixed.

Spoon into bowls and top with extra peanut butter, and the nuts and coconut. Serve immediately.

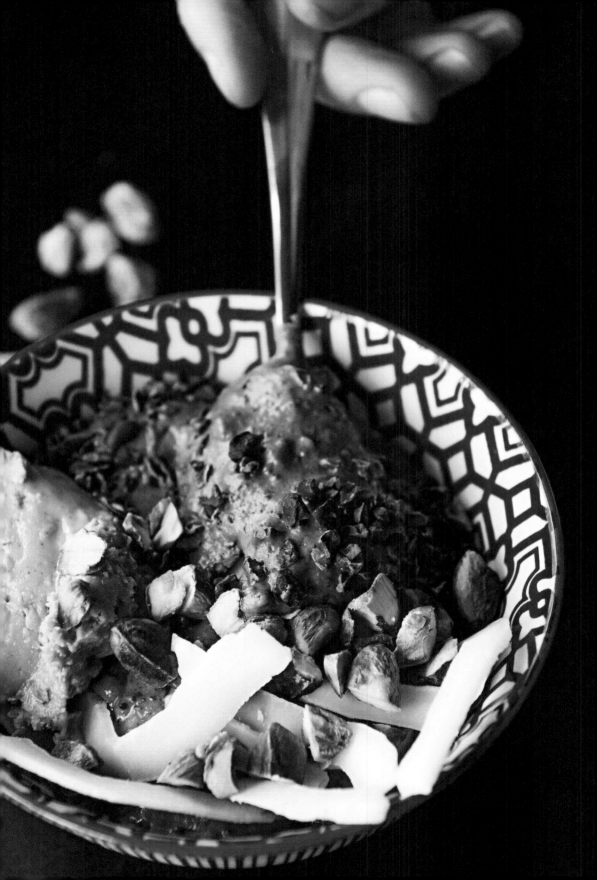

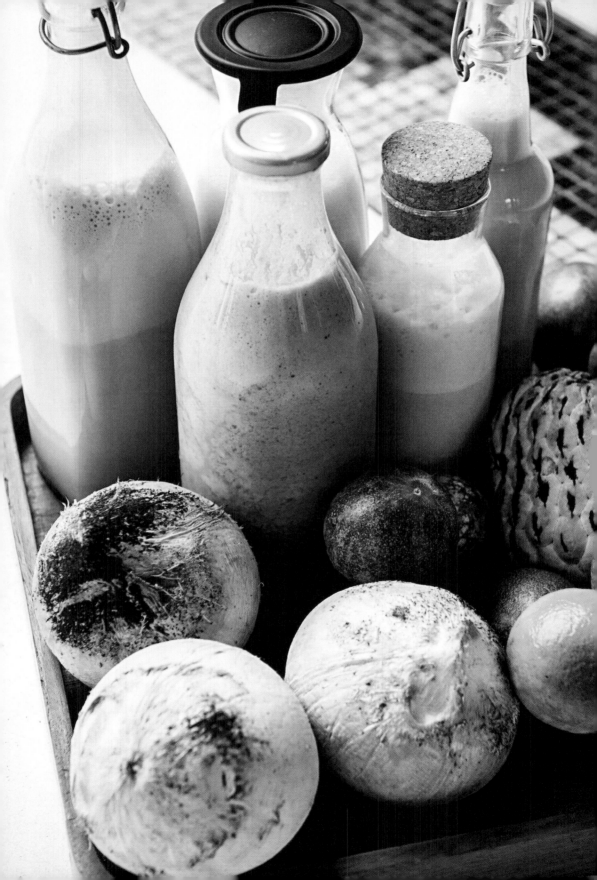

Raspberry and acai smoothie with whipped coconut

A ridiculously delicious smoothie that actually works both as a dessert and for breakfast. The whipped coconut cream makes it extra creamy.

SERVES 4

4 ripe bananas, peeled, cut into chunks and frozen
100g/3½ oz/scant 1 cup raspberries, frozen
2 tsp acai powder
100ml/3½ fl oz/generous ⅓ cup nut milk of your choice
1 recipe quantity of Vanilla Coconut Cream (see page 98), chilled
2 tsp coconut sugar
½ tsp ground cinnamon

Put the frozen bananas, frozen raspberries, acai and nut milk in a blender and blend on the highest speed for a couple of minutes until thick and smooth. Pour into a bowl.

Rinse out the blender and blend the coconut cream, coconut sugar and cinnamon until smooth. Pour the mixture over the raspberry smoothie.

Stir a few times with a plastic or wooden spoon and pour into a clean bottle or 4 glasses. Enjoy straight away.

Back row: Chocolate and Hazelnut Milk, Oat Milk, Pistachio and Spirulina Milk. Front row: Raspberry and Acai Smoothie, Cardamom Nut Milk

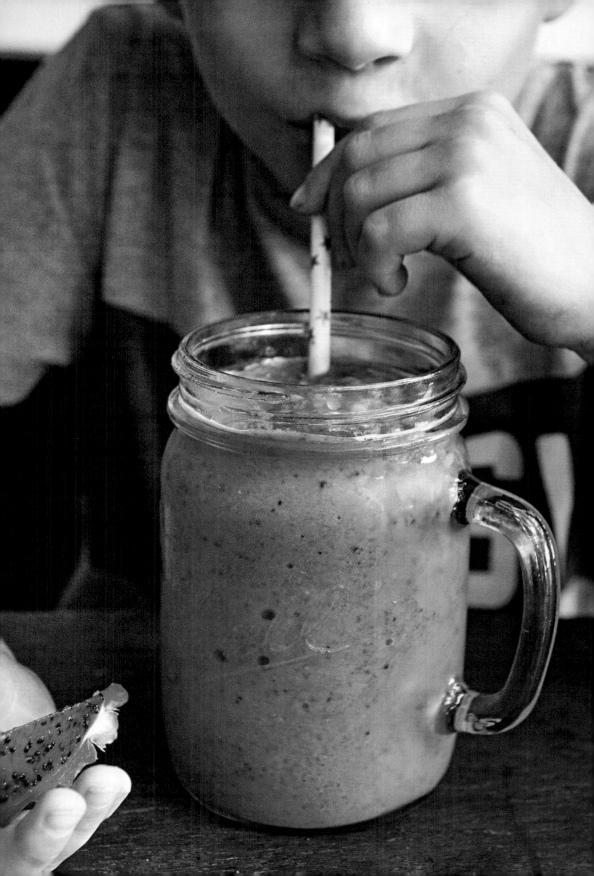

Dragon fruit smoothie

Dragon fruit, or pitaya, is not only nutritious, it's also colourful and fun to add to smoothies.

SERVES 1

200ml/7fl oz/scant 1 cup Coconut Milk (see page 67)
½ dragon fruit, peeled, cut into chunks and frozen
1 ripe banana, peeled, cut into chunks and frozen
1 tsp acai powder
¼ tsp vanilla powder

TOPPING:

1 passion fruit, cut in half and fruit scooped out

Put all the ingredients in a blender and blend on the highest speed for 1 minute until smooth and creamy.

Pour into a glass and top with the passion fruit pulp. Serve immediately.

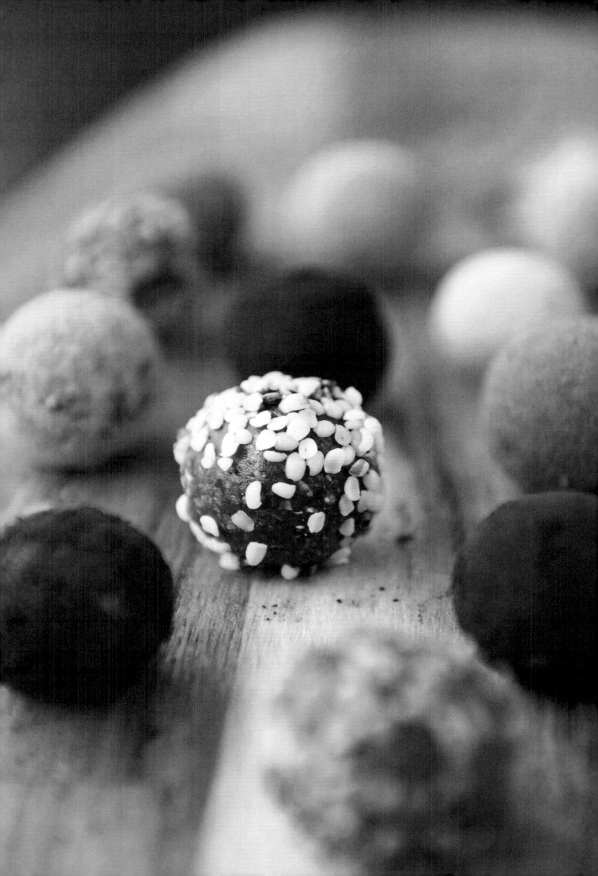

Energy balls

These energy balls are quick to make, taste like a treat, are jam-packed with nutrients and are easy to bring with you. This makes a handy base recipe, but do experiment with different flavourings. Try serving them with a glass of nut milk or a bowl of dairy-free yogurt.

MAKES ABOUT 15

20 medjool dates, pitted and chopped
200g/7oz/1½ cups porridge oats (rolled oats)
2 tbsp cacao powder
1 tsp carob powder
½ tbsp ashwagandha powder
3 tbsp coconut oil, melted
a pinch of pink Himalayan salt

COATING:

beetroot (beet) powder
wheatgrass or chlorella powder
bee pollen
hemp protein powder

Put all the ingredients for the balls in a blender and blend until they come together into a lump of dough. Shape into 15 balls and roll in the superfood coating of your choice.

Leave the balls to firm up in the fridge for about 20 minutes before eating. Store in an airtight container in the fridge for up to 4 days.

TIP
A couple of balls before or during exercise will give a quick energy boost.

Coconut and hemp protein biscuits

These cookies are perfect for when you need a pick-me-up such as after exercise, or for kids if they need an energy boost.

MAKES ABOUT 8 SANDWICHED COOKIES

200g/7oz/2⅔ cups desiccated (shredded) coconut

4 tbsp sunflower seeds

1 tbsp psyllium husk

3 tbsp water

6 tbsp hemp protein powder

6 tbsp maple syrup

1 tsp vanilla powder

1 tsp ground cinnamon

a pinch of sea salt

a little coconut oil, melted (you may not need this)

FILLING:

1 recipe quantity of Vanilla Coconut Cream (see page 98)

Preheat the oven to 150°C/300°F/Gas Mark 2.

Put the coconut and sunflower seeds in a food processor and pulse until coarsely chopped. Tip into a large bowl.

Stir the psyllium husk into the water and leave to stand for 15 minutes or until it becomes egg-like in consistency. Add to the bowl with the rest of the ingredients and mix well. If the mixture is too crumbly, add a little coconut oil to bring it all together.

Place tablespoonfuls of the cookie mixture spaced apart on a large baking tray (sheet) lined with baking (parchment) paper – the mixture should make about 16 cookies. Flatten the cookies into evenly-sized rounds using the back of the spoon. Bake for 15 minutes or until evenly golden in colour. Leave to cool on the tray.

When the cookies have cooled, turn half of them over, bottom-side up, and place a spoonful of the coconut cream on top. Place the remaining cookies on top as lids.

Serve immediately or store in an airtight container in the fridge for 4–5 days.

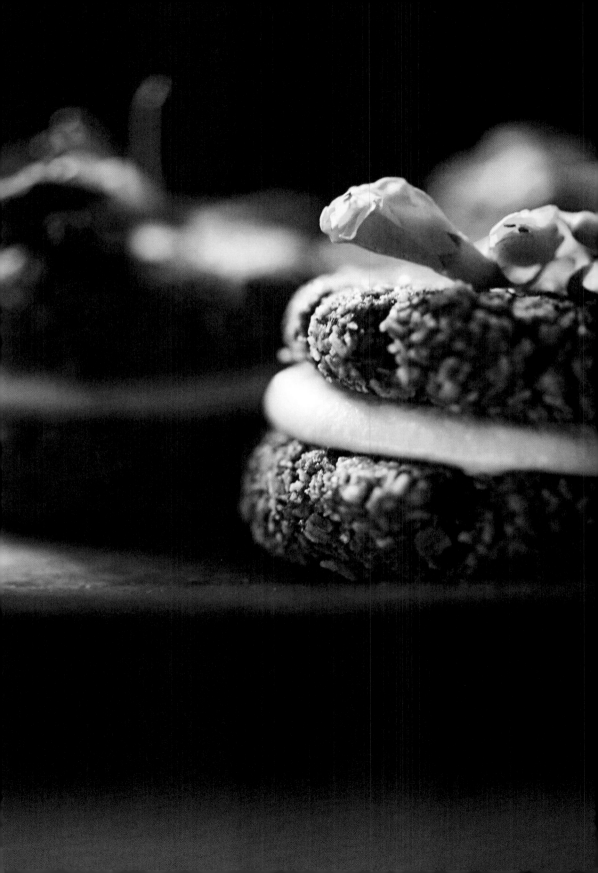

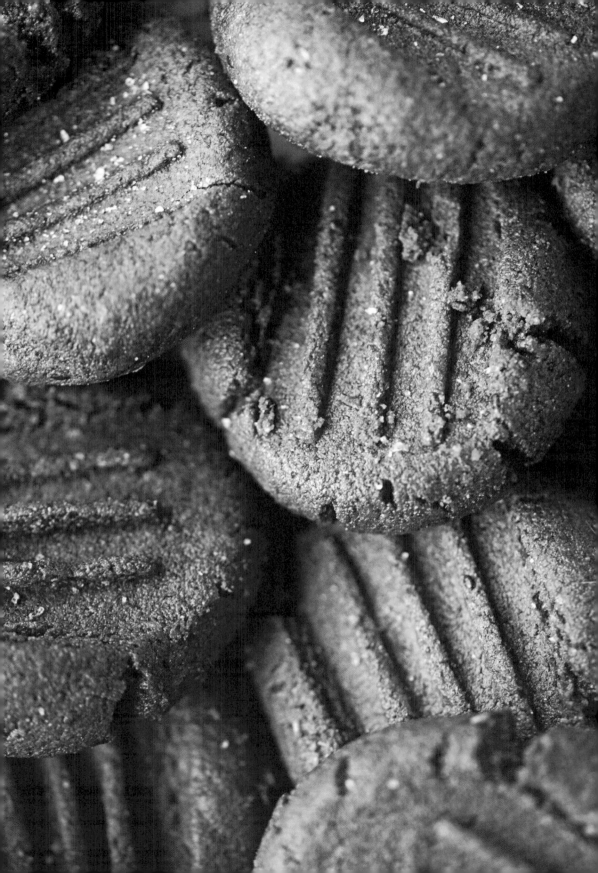

Spicy almond butter biscuits

For this recipe, I use teff flour, which is made from ground grass seeds. Teff is naturally gluten free and is rich in protein and minerals such as magnesium, phosphorus, iron and zinc, as well as being a good source of fibre. You can replace the almond butter with macadamia butter, if you prefer.

MAKES ABOUT 20

325g/11½ oz/2⅔ cups teff flour
½ tsp sea salt, plus extra for sprinkling
½ tsp ground cinnamon
375g/13oz Almond Butter (see page 29)
200ml/7fl oz/scant 1 cup maple syrup
200ml/7fl oz/scant 1 cup cold-pressed coconut oil, melted
½ tsp vanilla powder
¼ tsp ground ginger

Preheat the oven to 175°C/350°F/Gas Mark 4.

Mix together the flour, salt and cinnamon in a bowl. Add the almond butter, syrup, coconut oil, vanilla and ginger. Mix thoroughly until combined into a ball of dough.

Roll the dough into 20 small balls and place them spaced apart on a large baking tray (sheet) lined with baking (parchment) paper. Carefully flatten the balls using the back of a fork. Sprinkle the tops with a little extra salt.

Bake the biscuits for 10 minutes until crisp and golden. Leave to cool on a wire rack.

Serve immediately or store in an airtight container for 4–5 days.

Caramel sauce two ways

Both these sauces are equally delicious. The date caramel is quicker to make and it's good to have a jar at hand for feeding a milk kefir or to sweeten bread, vegan desserts, sauces or cream. Coconut caramel works perfectly with dairy-free ice cream or for sweetening yogurt.

Date caramel paste

MAKES 1 SMALL JAR

20–25 medjool dates, pitted and chopped

Put the dates in a food processor. Add a splash of water and blend until the dates are smooth and creamy in consistency.

Spoon into a clean jar with a tight-fitting lid. Store in the fridge and use within 2 weeks.

Coconut caramel

MAKES 200 ML/7 FL OZ/ SCANT 1 CUP

400ml/14fl oz/1¾ cups Vanilla Coconut Cream (see page 98)

210g/7½ oz/heaped 1 cup coconut sugar

½ tsp vanilla powder

a pinch of sea salt

Bring the coconut cream and sugar to the boil in a small pan. Turn the heat down and leave to simmer on a low heat for 15 minutes or until the mixture thickens.

Remove the pan from the heat and stir in the vanilla and salt. Leave to cool.

Pour into a clean jar with a tight-fitting lid. Store in the fridge and use within 5 days.

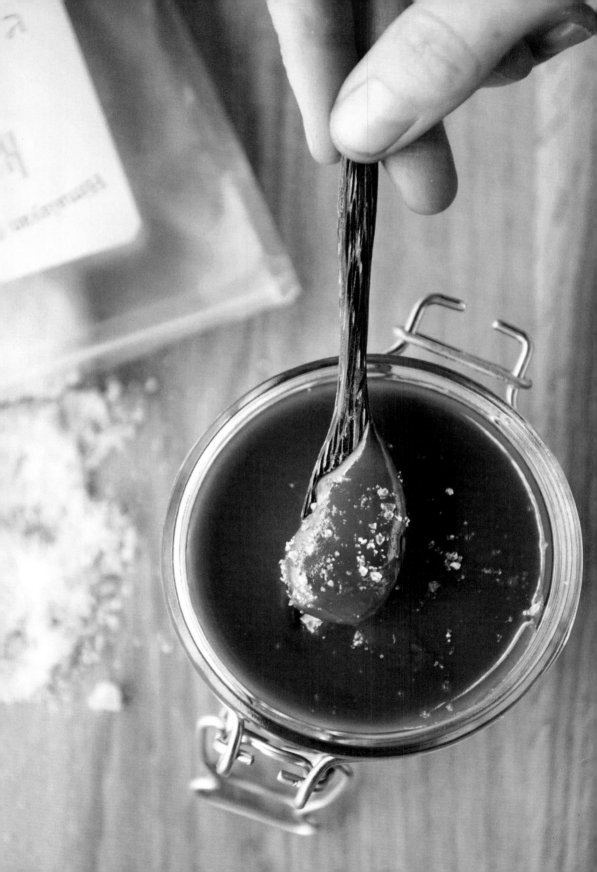

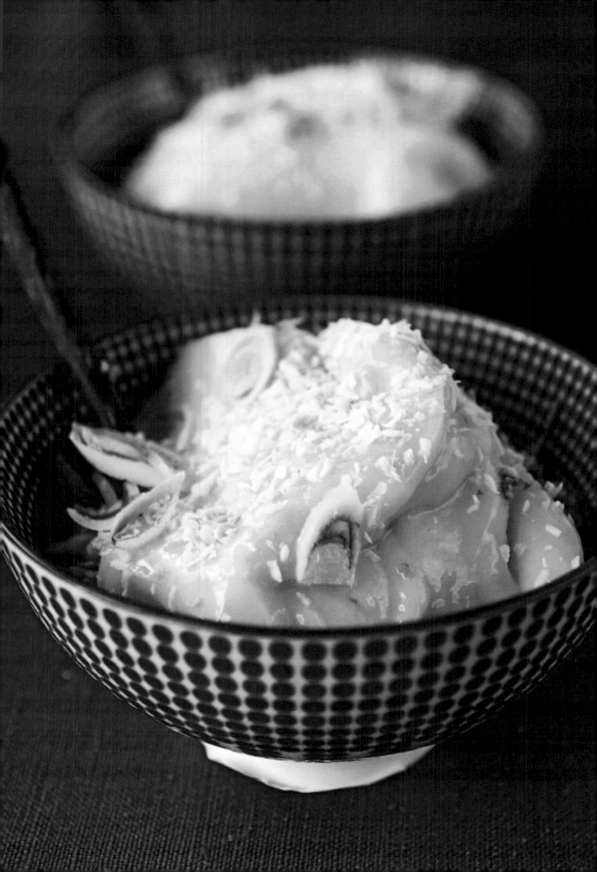

Yogurt ice cream
with mango, lime and coconut

Ripe mango is perfect in ice cream since it is naturally sweet and becomes creamy when blended. Add coconut water to the mixture, if you want to make a smoothie instead.

SERVES 2-4

2 tbsp desiccated (shredded) coconut
240g/8½ oz/generous 1 cup Coconut Yogurt
(see page 90)
juice and finely grated zest of 1 lime
250g/9oz/1½ cups frozen mango chunks

Toast the coconut in a dry frying pan (skillet) on a medium-low heat until light golden. Set aside and leave to cool.

Put the yogurt, lime juice and frozen mango in a food processor and blend until smooth and creamy.

Pour the mixture into a freezerproof container. Put it in the freezer and freeze, stirring the ice cream two or three times every 40 minutes to break up the ice crystals, until frozen.

About 20 minutes before serving, remove the ice cream from the freezer to soften slightly. Serve it topped with the toasted coconut and lime zest.

Nut biscuits

You can use whichever leftover nut pulp you've got to hand for this recipe, but it should preferably still be moist. Add a tablespoon or two of water to the dough if the pulp has dried out.

MAKES ABOUT 20

1 tbsp coconut oil, melted
1 tbsp Almond Butter (see page 29)
2 tbsp maple syrup
175g/6oz/scant 1 cup pulp from making nut milk
50g/1¾ oz/½ cup ground almonds
1 tbsp cacao powder
a little sea salt
1 tbsp cacao nibs
1 tbsp chopped sunflower seeds

Preheat the oven to 180°C/350°F/ Gas Mark 4.

Mix the coconut oil, almond butter and maple syrup together in a bowl. Add the rest of the ingredients, except cacao nibs and sunflower seeds. When the dough is evenly mixed, stir in the nibs and seeds.

Roll the dough into 20 small balls and place them spaced apart on a large baking tray (sheet) lined with baking (parchment) paper. Flatten the balls slightly using the back of a fork.

Bake the biscuits for 10–12 minutes until crisp and golden.

Leave to cool on a wire rack. Store in an airtight container and eat within 3–4 days.

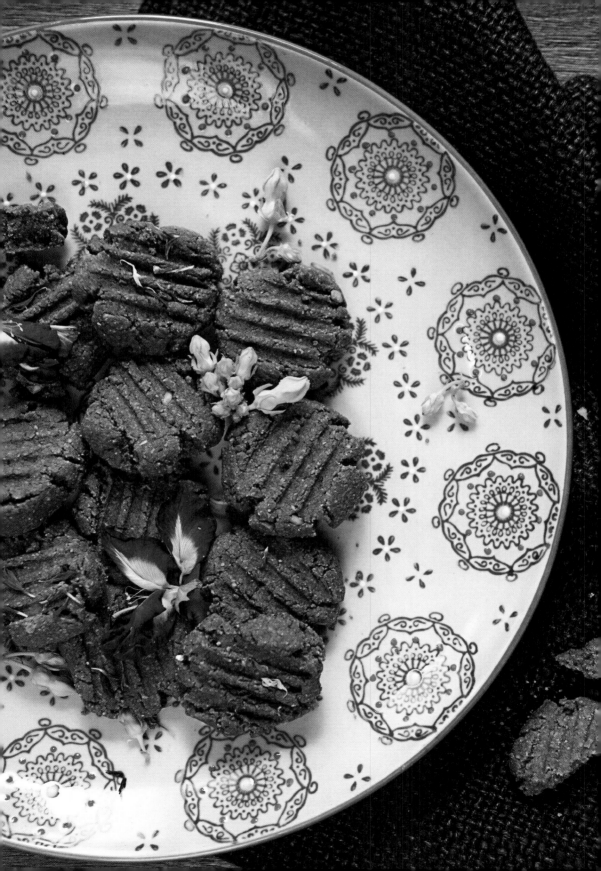

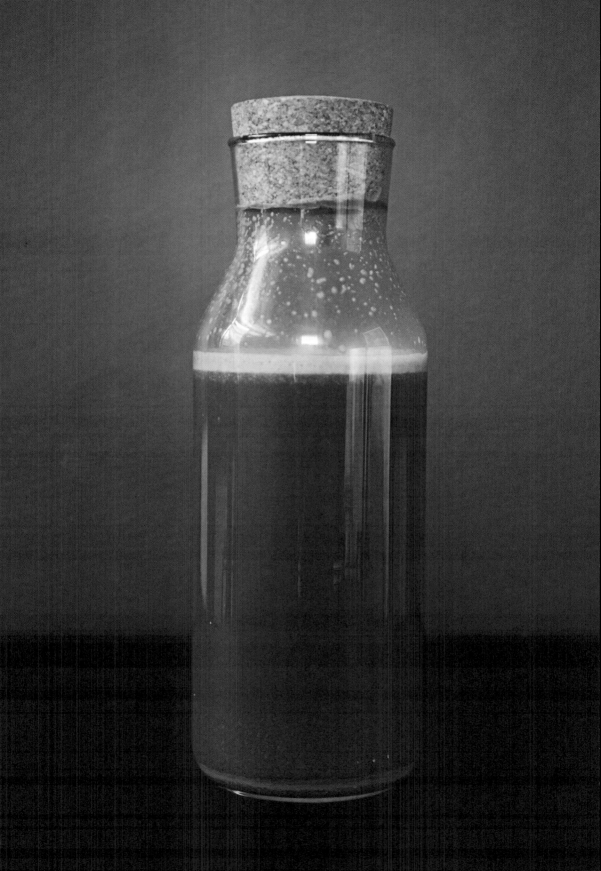

Spirulina and coconut milk

This is perfect if you want a ready-mixed drink in the morning for breakfast, or it can be used as a base for a smoothie or smoothie bowl. Spirulina is a superfood, a type of blue-green algae that is rich in chlorophyll, which the cells in our body like. It's also rich in B vitamins and protein, so it's a valuable source of nutrients, especially for vegetarians and vegans.

SERVES ABOUT 2

500ml/18fl oz/generous 2 cups Coconut Milk (see page 67)

2–3 tsp spirulina powder

1 tsp maca or ginseng powder

Put all the ingredients in a blender and blend on the highest speed for 1 minute until smooth. Pour into a clean bottle with a tight-fitting lid.

Store in the fridge and use within 2 days.

Smoothie bowl

SERVES 2

2–3 large ripe bananas, peeled, cut into chunks and frozen

1 recipe quantity of Spirulina and Coconut Milk (see above)

a handful of baby spinach leaves

fresh fruit and nuts, to serve

Put all the ingredients in a blender and blend on the highest speed for 2 minutes or until smooth and creamy.

Pour into 2 bowls and serve topped with fresh fruit and nuts.

Berry milk
with reishi and acai

Reishi, also called lingzhi mushroom, is an adaptogenic that boosts the immune system. Here, it's combined with almond milk and acai powder, the latter being rich in antioxidants, to make this blueberry milk. It's the perfect start to the day and is delicious with porridge or in a smoothie.

SERVES ABOUT 2

500ml/18fl oz/generous 2 cups Almond Milk (see page 59)

1 tsp blueberry powder

1 tsp acai powder

1 tsp reishi powder

½ tsp vanilla powder

Put all the ingredients in a blender and blend on the highest speed for 1 minute until smooth. Pour into a clean bottle with a tight-fitting lid.

Store in the fridge and use within 2 days.

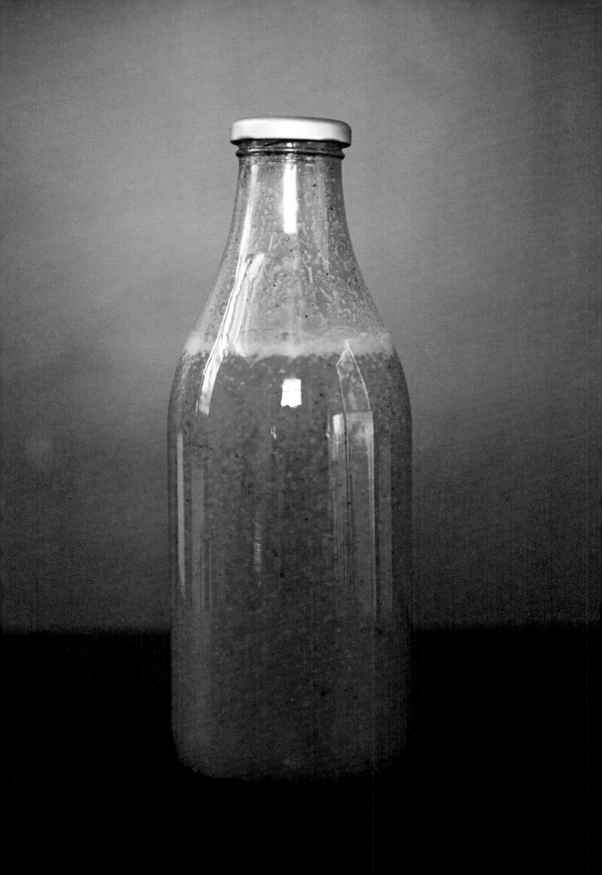

INDEX

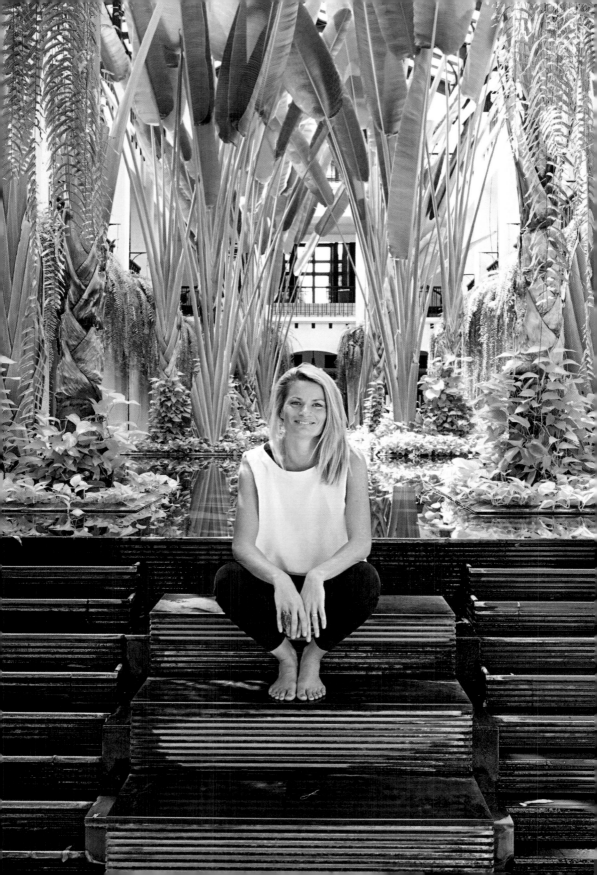

Thank you

To my publisher Johanna Kullman and Norstedts who believe in my idea and vision for a greener future!

To my children who have given me more patience than I ever thought I was capable of and who also give me such an incredible amount of happiness and love in life.

To my husband who, in turn, has showed that he is patient with me and who supports me through good times and bad so that I can fulfil my dreams. Thanks Henrik!

To Maria Selin for patiently sending the manuscript back and forth in search of the right tone of language.

To Sanna Sporrong who is my designer. Thanks for designing the book of my dreams and for going all the way with your creativity.

Thanks to Jason Lang, my photographer/restaurateur/entrepreneur, in whom I've found a good friend.

Thank you The Siam, the most beautiful hotel Bangkok has to offer, for giving us the opportunity and trust to take pictures on your amazing property.

To Bagaren och Kocken and Blendtec. I wouldn't have managed for all the tea in China without the strong motor in my machine.

To Granit for always being kind to me and for lending me your nice things.

And last but absolutely not least, to you who are now reading my book. I love this book as if it were my fourth baby and hope it will be of great use to you.

For any recipe that you try, please share! #vegandairy

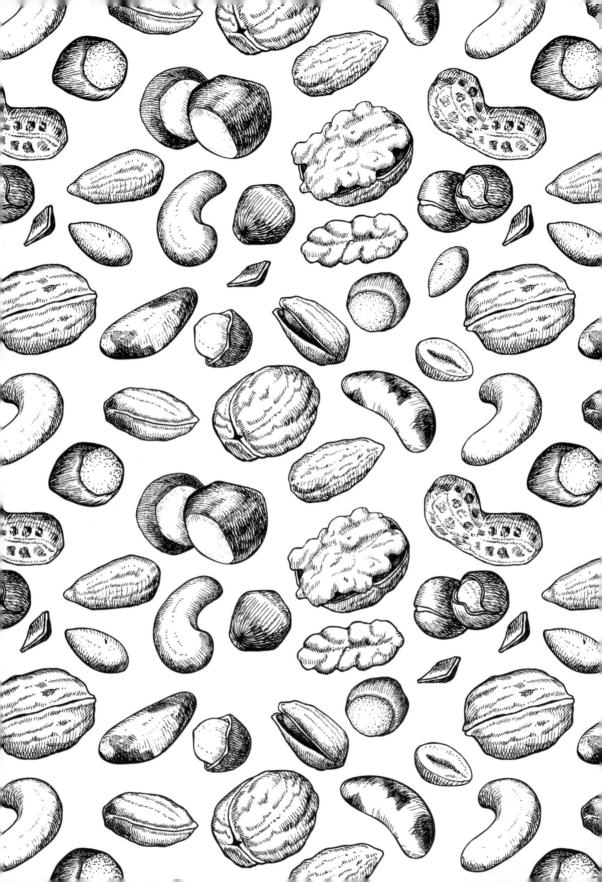